Essentials of Nonprescription Medications and Devices

Essentials of Nonprescription Medications and Devices

Elaine D Mackowiak BS Pharm, MS, PhD, RPh
Professor, Department of Pharmacy Practice, Temple University,
Philadelphia, PA, USA

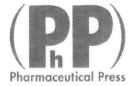

Pharmaceutical Press

To my children Jeffrey and Lisa, who had to tolerate my frequent late days and evenings due to work related responsibilities. To my late husband, Robert, and my parents, Veronica and the late Stanley De Cusatis, for their encouragement in all my endeavors.

Published by the Pharmaceutical Press
An imprint of RPS Publishing

© Pharmaceutical Press 2010

(**PP**) is a trade mark of RPS Publishing

RPS Publishing is the publishing organisation of the Royal Pharmaceutical Society of Great Britain

First published 2010
Reprinted 2014

Typeset by Thomson Digital, Noida, India
Printed in Great Britain by TJ International, Padstow, Cornwall

ISBN 978 0 85369 861 6

A catalogue record for this book is available from the British Library.

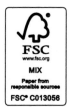

FSC
www.fsc.org
MIX
Paper from
responsible sources
FSC® C013056

Contents

Preface

There is a large increase in the number of people assuming more responsibility for their own healthcare by using nonprescription medications, especially for many common conditions such as colds, allergies, and heartburn. Two important factors contribute to this rise in self-care. First, the number of prescription (Rx) drugs that have been switched to over-the-counter (OTC) status (Rx–OTC switch) by the Food and Drug Administration (FDA) has increased, making more effective medications available to consumers at reduced costs. Second, the increased cost of medical care has prompted many people to go without medical insurance, thus avoiding or delaying a visit to a physician.

Self-care may involve better nutrition, more physical activity, and use of nonprescription drug products. Several different types of product are available, including home test kits and medical devices, OTC drugs, dietary supplements and herbal remedies, and homeopathic products. There are important distinctions among these products that pharmacists and consumers should understand before choosing a product for use.

This text is intended to provide pharmacists, pharmacy students, and individuals interested in self-care an easy to use reference for common conditions and products available for prevention and treatment. The initial chapter of this text describes the role the FDA exercises in controlling and monitoring products for self-care in the USA. The chapters that follow provide brief descriptions of common medical conditions amenable to self-care for specific physiological systems and nonprescription products available for treatment.

Drug therapy discussions are based on the specific pharmacological categories of nonprescription products approved by the FDA through either its monograph system for OTC drugs or its Rx–OTC switch program. Popular dietary supplements, herbal products, and homeopathic products are discussed when appropriate. The format for each chapter includes the pharmacological drug category of the drug for therapy, indications for use, the mode of action of the drug, warnings and precautions for the drug's use, recommended dose, and popular brand name products available in the USA. Sample case scenarios are included at the end of the chapter.

Elaine D Mackowiak
September, 2009

Elaine D Mackowiak practiced briefly as a hospital pharmacist but has over 40 years of experience as a community pharmacist in both independent and chain pharmacies. She joined the faculty of Temple University School of Pharmacy in 1964 and has taught in ambulatory care and nonprescription pharmacy courses for 35 years. She served as Chairperson of the Department of Pharmacy Practice for 8 years. She has taught in the nuclear pharmacy program since its inception, and became Director of the Nuclear Pharmacy program in 1975, a position she continues to hold.

Her publications and presentations include the areas of nonprescription medications, pharmaceutical education, medication management in geriatric populations, nuclear pharmacy, radiation safety, diagnostic imaging drugs, and health hazards of base metals in dental student populations.

She is a member of the American Pharmacists Association (Academy of Pharmacy Practice and Nuclear Pharmacy), American Association of Colleges of Pharmacy, the Health Physics Society, Sigma Xi, Rho Chi National Honor Society, and Lambda Kappa Sigma Professional Pharmacy Fraternity.

Acknowledgments

The author thanks Ms Barbara Grissani, BA, technical support specialist, for her friendship and assistance in preparation of this manuscript and many other manuscripts over the years. The author thanks Albert Wertheimer, PhD, Professor of Pharmacy Economics, for his encouragement during this endeavor.

1

Regulation of the nonprescription drug market by the US Food and Drug Administration

The US drug marketing system

Drug safety

In 1938, there was a major revision of the Food, Drug and Cosmetic Act of 1906 (FD&C), which formed the foundation for the current authority in regulating drugs held by the Food and Drug Administration (FDA). One major provision of the Act required manufacturers to submit to the FDA information for all new drugs that provided proof of their safety in order to be approved for marketing. Drugs used before the 1938 revision are not new drugs and remain in the marketplace as GRAS (generally recognized as safe) drugs, provided there is no substantial change in their formulations, recommended doses, or use.[1]

Prescription and nonprescription drugs

There was no clear legal distinction between prescription (Rx) and nonprescription drugs until the passage of the Durham–Humphrey Amendments in 1951. The amendments required all drugs that are habit forming or have potentially severe toxicity to carry a printed statement on the label, known as the Rx legend. The statement or legend is: 'Caution: Federal law prohibits dispensing without a prescription.'[1] Drug products not fitting this description do not have the statement on their labels and are known as 'nonlegend' or over-the-counter (OTC) drugs.

Drug efficacy

The Kefauver–Harris amendments of the 1938 FD&C Act in 1962 required manufacturers to submit information proving the efficacy (effectiveness) of a new drug as well as safety data in order to be approved by the FDA.[1] The amendments included all drugs approved between 1938 and 1962, for which data had to be submitted to prove their efficacy in order for the drug to remain in the marketplace. This review process became the Drug Efficacy Study Implementation program (DESI).

However, the many drugs in use before 1938 that had GRAS status were not reviewed, creating the GRAE (generally recognized as effective) status. The majority of dietary supplements, herbal remedies, and homeopathic products are GRASE drugs (generally recognized as safe and effective). If manufacturers of GRASE products change formulations, recommended doses and/or intended use, the FDA considers these products to be new, unapproved drugs. Since the manufacturers had not submitted a new drug application (NDA) for their product, the FDA issues a guidance document discussing how it intends to implement its policy for removing these marketed but unapproved products from the marketplace.[2]

Nonprescription or OTC drugs

FDA's monograph process

The DESI program involved all drugs with the exception of GRASE products, and the FDA decided to review all the prescription drugs before beginning a review of OTC drugs. This process began in 1972 with the creation of panels of experts that reviewed OTC individual drugs or ingredients within a therapeutic drug category. The panels published their reports to the FDA in the *Federal Register*, identifying OTC drugs, active ingredients, determined to be safe and effective and those that were not safe for OTC use. Some OTC drugs deemed to be safe did not have sufficient evidence to prove efficacy. These drugs were placed in a temporary category that allowed them to remain in the marketplace while manufacturers were granted more time to submit data to prove efficacy. All panels have submitted their reports.[1–3]

The FDA reviews each panel's report and publishes an Advanced Notice of Rulemaking in the *Federal Register* where all subsequent FDA actions are reported. The FDA invites comments on its proposed rules, reviews them, and publishes a Proposed Rule or Tentative Final Monograph. After another comment period, the FDA publishes a Final Rule or Final Monograph. All OTC drugs that have proved safety and efficacy are known as monograph drugs. Any drug that is unsafe or remains in the temporary category (requiring more information to prove efficacy) becomes a non-monograph drug once the Final Monograph is published. Unsafe drugs must be removed from the marketplace. A drug that has not proved efficacy cannot appear on the label as an active ingredient but may remain in the product and must appear in the inactive ingredient.[1,2]

The OTC review process is quite long, and a few therapeutic categories of drugs remain in the Proposed Rule or Tentative Final Monograph stage at this time (2009). Monographs for OTC drugs contain the following information: list of approved active ingredients, dosage formulations, recommended doses, required labeling information, packaging information, and/or testing information for some products. Some monographs also contain labeling information for use of the active ingredients by healthcare professionals. If a manufacturer wishes to market a drug in a monograph, no prior approval from the FDA is needed if all the requirements in the monograph are followed and if current good manufacturing practices are followed.[1,2]

New OTC drug process

A new OTC drug may enter the market if the FDA approves an NDA submitted by the manufacturer, or if the manufacturer submits a supplemental NDA for an Rx–OTC switch product. If the Rx–OTC switch process is followed, the FDA may grant the manufacturer from one to three years of exclusivity for marketing the product, but it may also grant no exclusivity.[1,2] Once the exclusivity period has expired, another manufacturer may submit an NDA to the FDA for approval if it wished to market the drug. If the FDA places the drug in a monograph at some time after the exclusivity period expires, a manufacturer must follow the monograph information if it wished to market the drug and it does not have to file an NDA.

OTC product labels

If a product's label cannot provide sufficient information for the public to use the product safely, or if the condition for its use cannot be self-determined and/or self-monitored, the product will not become an OTC drug. The OTC drug labels must include the following information: name of active ingredient(s), intended use of the product, warnings or precautions, potential adverse effects and/or potential drug interactions, directions for use (dose and frequency of administration based on age or weight), proper storage information, and list of inactive ingredients. All products also have an expiration date.

All OTC drugs contain the following warnings:

1   do not use the product if the individual is allergic to the ingredient(s) in the product;
2   do not use the product if a woman is pregnant without the advice of her physician;
3   do not use the product if a woman is breast feeding without the advice of her physician; and
4   keep the product and all medication out of the reach of children.

Most OTC products are not recommended for use in children under 2 years of age without the advice of a physician or healthcare professional.

OTCs available from pharmacists only

Nearly all OTC drugs are available in any retail store in the US. However, federal law restricts the sale of OTC drugs that have a potential for abuse, such as codeine cough syrups and pseudoephedrine, to sale from pharmacies.[1,4] An individual must provide identification and proof of age and sign a form that the pharmacist is required to maintain of these sales. Because there is significant abuse of dextromethorphan, a cough suppressant, by adolescents, it may be included in this category in the near future. Individual states may have more restrictive pharmacy laws than the federal law, and the reader should become aware of the laws in the states where they reside; for example, the Commonwealth of Pennsylvania requires a prescription for all cough medications containing codeine.

Other drugs may also be restricted to sales by pharmacists. When the FDA approved Plan B, the emergency contraceptive drug, as an OTC drug, it became available only from the pharmacist.[5] Products restricted to sale by a pharmacist may be considered to be behind-the-counter (BTC) drugs but this is not an official FDA drug category at this time.

OTCs for physician-diagnosed and chronic conditions

Although most OTC drugs are used for self-diagnosed, self-limiting conditions, there are exceptions. An example is the use of OTC vaginal antifungal drugs. If a woman had a previous vaginal candida (yeast) infection that was diagnosed by a physician and the problem recurs, she may self-treat with OTC drugs.

Another example is the use of OTC bronchodilating drugs. These products are to be used only if a physician has diagnosed an individual with asthma and the asthma is not a self-limiting condition.

OTC drugs are recommended for a specific period of time and all labels contain statements advising individuals to see a healthcare professional if symptoms are not relieved or have worsened within the recommended period of use.

Relationship of OTC drug's active ingredient content and brand name

Manufacturers of OTC products may change the active ingredient without a change being made in the product's name. Kaopectate, a product used to treat diarrhea, is an excellent example of this situation. The original Kaopectate product contained kaolin and pectin as active ingredients. The final monograph for antidiarrheal products concluded that neither was effective and they were declared non-monograph drugs. The manufacturer reformulated the product so that it contained attapulgite, which was classified as a monograph drug. A revision of the final monograph for antidiarrheal drugs by the FDA reclassified attapulgite as non-monograph and bismuth subsalicylate as a monograph antidiarrheal. The present Koapectate product contains bismuth subsalicylate. Therefore, an individual must read the labels carefully when purchasing OTC drugs. This situation could never happen with prescription drugs, because once a drug is given a brand name, the ingredient cannot be changed.

Brand name and extended products

Manufacturers that have very successful brand name products which have established brand loyalty among the public will market new products that include the brand name but have different active ingredients. For example, Dramamine, a product that is used for preventing and treating motion sickness, has always contained dimenhydrinate as its active ingredient. The manufacturer markets Dramamine Less Drowsy, also a product that is used for motion sickness, but containing meclizine. Another example is the popular antacid Mylanta. As a suspension, this product contains aluminum hydroxide and magnesium hydroxide, but as Children's Mylanta tablets, it contains calcium carbonate.

This situation is very confusing for both pharmacists and the public since ingredient changes can be so easily altered by manufacturers. Product labels should be read carefully by everyone purchasing or recommending an OTC product for use.

Cost of OTC drugs

Manufacturers tend to price their products in a manner that is competitive with other similar products. Popular brand name products must compete with generic formulations of OTC products that are less expensive, in the same manner as prescription drugs. If there are significant differences in costs among products used for the same purpose, it is noted in the discussion here. For example, electronic digital fever thermometers cost less than $10.00, but infrared devices cost $35.00 or more. (Prices obtained from the internet; www.drugstore.com)

Dietary supplements

Dietary supplements, primarily vitamins and herbal products, are not OTC drugs because they are GRASE products and their manufacturers do not have to prove safety and efficacy for them to remain in the marketplace. It is the responsibility of the FDA to prove that a GRASE product is not safe in order for it to be removed from the marketplace.

Specific information for regulation and sale of these products appears in the Dietary Supplement and Education Act of 1994 (DSHEA).[6] The labels for these products must contain the following statements: 'This product has not been evaluated by the Food and Drug Administration.' 'This product is not intended to diagnose, treat, cure or prevent any disease.'

The popularity of dietary supplements has grown in the last several years, prompting the National Institutes of Health to establish a new division, the National Institute on Complementary Alternative Medicine. The Institute has sponsored several clinical trials of popular supplements for treating common conditions such as the common cold, osteoarthritis, and several other common ailments. These trials have failed to establish efficacy for these products at this time.

Homeopathic drugs

Certain homeopathic drugs that are claimed to treat a serious disease were included in the 1938 FD&C Act and require a prescription by a homeopathic physician. However, many homeopathic products are available OTC and the labels for these must contain the statements: 'This product has not been evaluated by the Food and Drug Administration.' 'This product is not intended to diagnose, treat, cure or prevent any disease.'

Homeopathy, an alternative medical practice, employs three basic principles. First, the ingredient used to treat an ailment should cause the same symptoms as the individual's complaint (like treats like); for example, a drug that causes nausea should be used to treat individuals who complain of nausea. Second, the ingredient should be as dilute as possible. Third, a process of shaking must occur between dilutions (succussion). Homeopathic theory states that succussion imparts an imprint in the solutions that increases its effectiveness.[7,8] Neither the American Medical Association nor the American Pharmaceutical Association accept homeopathy as conventional therapy at this time.

Information on the label of a homeopathic product differs from that appearing on labels of OTC drugs or dietary supplements. The label of a homeopathic product must contain the ingredient list, directions for use, indication for use, and the dilution used in producing the product. All dilutions are made from an original solution called the mother tincture. Dilutions are expressed in Arabic numbers and Roman numerals. The Roman numeral indicates the dilution, for example, X is a 1:10 dilution; C, a 1:100 dilution. The Arabic number indicates how many times the dilution is performed. For example, feverfew 3X on the label of a product means that a 1:10 dilution of a sample of feverfew from the mother tincture is made and shaken. This preparation is again diluted 1:10, shaken, and another 1:10 dilution is made, for a total of three dilutions.

The OTC drugs and dietary supplement labels list the quantity of drug in each tablet in units of mass or weight, such as grams (g) or milligrams (mg). Labels of liquid products list the amount of active ingredient as a concentration, weight per unit of volume, or milligram per teaspoonful (5 mL). The label of a homeopathic product does not provide the amount of drug in the mother tincture, so the amount of drug is not known.

Healthcare professionals are well aware of the positive effect that may be produced by a placebo, a formulation that contains no active ingredient. The extreme dilution of homeopathic products may allow them to fit a definition of placebo. This is one possible explanation for the efficacy attributed to homeopathic products. Because of this dilution process used in homeopathic products, very little drug is administered, which greatly reduces the possibility of adverse effects. Allergic reactions remain as the most significant adverse effect possible in sensitive individuals.

The pharmacist's role in self-care

When an individual consults a pharmacist about a medical problem, the first decision by the pharmacist is to determine whether or not the problem should be managed by self-care or should be referred to a physician. The pharmacist should obtain information from the individual about the current problem, including a description of the symptoms, the severity, onset, and duration of symptoms. The pharmacist should ask about any treatment or drug therapy the individual has tried and the success or failure of the treatment. The pharmacist should review the medical history and use of prescription and OTC drugs, dietary supplements, herbal products, and homeopathic products.

The pharmacist accesses this information and develops a self-care plan for the individual. This plan may include OTC drugs, dietary supplements, homeopathic drugs, ancillary therapy (a healthy diet and/or mild exercise program for weight loss), education and counseling, and follow-up monitoring of the individual. Effective communication between the pharmacist and the individual are essential for a successful outcome to result from their interaction.

Important sources of OTC drug information

National phone number for Poison Control: 1–800–222–1222.

Reporting adverse drug effects: https://www.accessdata.fda.gov/scripts/medwatch/medwatch_online.cfm.

Reporting adverse vaccine effects: www.vaers.hhs.gov.

General medical information: www.webmd.com; www.mayoclinic.com.

General medication safety information: www.consumermedsafety.org/.

National Center for Complementary and Alternative Medicine (NCCAM): nccam.nih.gov.

Natural Medicine Comprehensive Database: www.naturalmedicine.com.

FDA center for Drug Evaluation and Research: www.fda.gov/cder.
FDA Office of In Vitro Diagnostic Devices: www.fda.gov/cdrh/oivd/.

References

1. Pray WS. *A History of Nonprescription Product Regulations*. New York: Haworth Press, 2003.
2. *Frequently Asked Questions on the Regulatory Process of Over-the-Counter (OTC) Drugs*. www.fda.gov/cder/about/smallbiz/OTC_FAQ.htm (accessed October 28, 2008).
3. *Guidance for FDA Staff and Industry Marketed Unapproved Drugs-Compliance Policy Guide* Sec.440.100. www.fda.gov/cder/guidance/6911fnl.htm (accessed September 8, 2008).
4. *Legal Requirements for the Sale and Purchase of Drug Products Containing Pseudoephedrine, Ephedrine, and Phenylpropanolamine*. www.fda.gov/cder/news/methamphetamine. htm (accessed October 28, 2008).
5. *FDA Approves Over-the-Counter Access for Plan B for Women 18 and Older. Prescription Remains Required for Those 17 and Under*. www.fda.gov/bbs/topics/NEWS/2006/NEW01436.html (accessed October 28, 2008).
6. Dietary Supplement Health and Education Act of 1994, Public Law 103-417. www.fda.gov/opacom/laws/dshea.html (accessed October 28, 2008).
7. Stehlin I. *Homeopathy: Real Medicine or Empty Promises?* www.fda.gov/fdac/features/096_home.html (accessed October 29, 2008).
8. *Conditions Under Which Homeopathic Drugs May Be Marketed*. www.fda.gov/ora/compliance_ref/cpg/cpgdrg/cpg400-400.html (accessed October 29, 2008).

2

Diagnostic home test kits

The FDA amended the FD&C Act of 1938 in 1976 to include the following definition for devices: '...an instrument, apparatus, implement, machine, contrivance, implant, *in vitro* reagent, or other similar or related article, including any component, part, or accessory, which is: (1) recognized in the official National Formulary or the US Pharmacopeia, or any supplement to them; (2) intended for use in the diagnosis of disease or other conditions, or in the cure, mitigation, treatment or prevention of disease, in man or other animals; or (3) intended to affect the structure or any function of the body of man or other animals, and which does not achieve any of its principal intended purposes through chemical action within or on the body of man or other animals and which is not dependent upon being metabolized for achievement of any of its principal intended purposes.'[1]

An OTC home test kit must have proved that the device is able to produce reliable results which are accurate when used by the population for whom the test is intended before the FDA grants approval.[2] The test device must demonstrate sensitivity (test results are positive if the individual has the condition) and accuracy (test results are negative if the individual does not have the condition). An individual should be able to obtain the same results as a health professional who uses the test, and the test should have some method that indicates that the test is complete and has been performed correctly.

There are two types of OTC home test devices. One type gives the result of the test once the directions for its use have been completed, for example a blood glucose test meter. The other type of device requires the patient to follow directions for obtaining a biological sample (a drop of blood or a urine sample), which is then mailed to the manufacturer where a laboratory test is performed to obtain the test's result, for example a home test kit for the human immunodeficiency virus (HIV). The individual contacts the manufacturer at a specified time after returning the test to obtain the laboratory's result.

Congress, through the Health Care Financing Administration (HCFA), regulates laboratory testing for humans by an act known as the Clinical Laboratory Improvements Amendment (CLIA). CLIA-waived tests are intended for use by individuals who have the least amount of training in laboratory techniques. The FDA approves OTC home test kits that are CLIA waived, but all not CLIA-waived tests are approved by the FDA for OTC use. Potential errors in performing these tests are minimized, and even if an inaccurate result occurs, it will not immediately endanger the health of the individual. The greater the number of steps in the test's procedure, the more likely it is that an individual will make a mistake that could give an erroneous result.

OTC home test kits are sold in pharmacies, other retail outlets, and on the internet. Individuals should be cautious about purchasing test kits, especially on the internet, because many devices are not FDA approved and there is no way to determine their accuracy. The Office of In Vitro Diagnostic Devices (OIVD) maintains a database of home test kits approved by the FDA available at its website.[3] One disadvantage of this site is that it only provides dates of approval and does not have information about whether or not the kit is currently available in the marketplace.

Users of home test kits should be aware of several important factors regarding their use. First, it is important to be certain that the expiration date of the kit has not passed and that the kit has been stored under proper conditions. Reagents and other components of the kit may be subject to degradation when stored improperly. All directions for use of the test kit must be followed precisely in order to be sure that the result obtained is accurate. However, not every test result will be correct 100% of the time, even when tests are performed by skilled professionals. A second test should be done to confirm the initial result. No important healthcare decision should be made on the result of a single home test kit result. If the test result indicates a serious medical condition, the result should be reported to the individual's physician, who will seek to verify the result and make appropriate recommendations for treatment when it is necessary.

Blood pressure monitoring devices

Hypertension, or high blood pressure, is one of the most common medical conditions in the USA and is an indication of cardiovascular disease. It is a condition that rarely has any symptoms during its early stages and is detected only by measurement with a blood pressure monitoring device. Uncontrolled hypertension increases an individual's risk of stroke, heart attacks, and kidney disease. Many individuals diagnosed as having hypertension by their physician may want to monitor their blood pressure between visits to the physician by purchasing blood pressure devices.

If the blood pressure values measured on the home blood pressure differ from those taken in the physician's office, no changes to medications should be made by an individual unless directed to do so by the physician. The individual should take the home device with them on the next visit to the physician to check the device's reading with those taken during the visit. If the home reading is different, the monitor must be recalibrated.

Mode of action
An inflatable cuff connected to a meter is placed on the upper part of the arm over the brachial artery and is inflated. An individual using a stethoscope listens for the appearance of the pulse, the systolic blood pressure (pressure against the artery wall when the heart contracts), while the pressure in the cuff is slowly released. The disappearance of the pulse indicates the diastolic blood pressure (arterial pressure when the heart ventricles relax and fill with blood). Accepted values for normal blood pressure are a systolic reading of less than 120 and a diastolic reading of less than 80 mmHg.

Warnings and precautions
A healthcare provider must teach an individual how to use an aneroid blood pressure monitor properly. The individual must have adequate dexterity to release air slowly and adequate hearing to hear the sounds with the stethoscope. Aneroid devices usually require calibration yearly. Blood pressure cuffs are available in different sizes and the individual must use the appropriate cuff to obtain a valid blood pressure reading.

Electronic blood pressure monitors

Mode of action
An inflatable cuff connected to a device that automatically inflates and deflates and has sensors that measure the systolic and diastolic blood pressure, displaying the values as a digital readout. These devices also display the pulse rate. The devices are much easier to use than aneroid devices but may be less accurate.

Warnings and precautions
These devices are battery operated and require replacement of the batteries. Electronic blood pressure monitors are available for use on the upper arm, wrist or finger, but the wrist and finger devices tend to be less accurate than those using the upper arm for measurement.

Products
The following manufacturers make several different models of the aneroid and electronic monitors: Omron, HoMedics, Luminiscope, Duro-Med and Samsung.

Cholesterol tests

Elevated blood cholesterol levels are associated with an increase risk of cardiovascular disease. A more precise evaluation of an individual's risk may be determined by measuring low-density lipoprotein cholesterol, high-density lipoprotein cholesterol, and triglycerides, not just total cholesterol levels.

OTC home tests kits are available for measuring these various cholesterol parameters.

Total cholesterol tests

Mode of action
A finger stick sample of capillary blood is placed in the well of a device that contains a chromatographic stick impregnated with enzymes (cholesterol esterase and cholesterol oxidase). Capillary attraction draws the sample over the reagents, producing a color on a calibrated scale. The value from the calibrated scale is compared with a test chart and the total cholesterol value is read in milligrams per deciliter (mg/dL). Individuals are advised to consult a physician if the value exceeds 200 mg/dL.

Warnings and precautions
This test kit requires several timed steps that must be performed correctly to obtain an accurate result. No acetaminophen (Tylenol) should be taken within 4 hours of testing, and ingestion of 500 mg or more of ascorbic acid (vitamin C) must be avoided. Both of these drugs may cause a falsely low result during the test.[4]

Products
CholesTrak, Home Access Instant Cholesterol Test, First Check Home Cholesterol Test.

Cholesterol and lipid profile test card

Return mail test

Mode of action
A finger stick sample of capillary blood is placed on a test pad of a card and returned to the manufacturer for laboratory analysis. The test kit consists of a lancet, band-aid, test card with a code, and a return mailer. The individual calls a toll free telephone number in a prescribed number of days after the test and speaks with a trained counselor who provides the test's results and answers any questions the individual may have.

Product
BioSafe Cholesterol Test.

At home test

Mode of action
The device is a battery operated, photoreflectance meter that measures the intensity of color produced on a reagent strip containing a drop of capillary blood from a finger stick. The test result appears digitally on the meter. There

are three different types of strip, each with its own microchip, to determine total cholesterol, high-density lipoprotein cholesterol, and triglycerides. Directions provide information for the calculation of low-density lipoprotein cholesterol levels.

Products
CardioChek, Landmark Full Lipid Panel Cholesterol Test. This type of detector provides more complete information and is more costly ($125) than total cholesterol measurement kits, which cost less than $15.

Cholesterol and blood glucose meters

Mode of action
The device is a battery operated monitor that determines blood glucose levels and total cholesterol levels from a finger stick of capillary blood by using two different reagent strips.

Products
Accu-Chek Instant Plus, QSTEPS Biometer Dual Monitoring System.

Diabetes monitoring devices

Blood glucose monitors

Individuals who require injections of insulin (type 1 diabetes) must know the concentration of glucose in their blood in order to control their diabetes. Some individuals who have type 2 diabetes and control their diabetes with oral medications may also measure their blood glucose levels. Individuals with type 1 diabetes should measure blood glucose at least four times a day, and adjust the amount of insulin required based on these measurements. Lack of control of blood glucose increases the risk of cardiovascular disease, kidney disease, neuropathy, and visual impairment in individuals who have diabetes.

A small drop of capillary blood from a finger prick or an alternative site (upper arm or forearm, thigh or palm) is placed on a reagent strip inserted into a blood glucose monitor. Glucose reacts with the reagent strip, which contains an enzyme, producing an electrochemical reaction. A biosensor in the monitor converts the electrical signal to a digital value that displays the concentration of glucose as milligrams per deciliter (mg/dL).

Accurate results depend on the following conditions:

• the meter is clean and calibrated if necessary (some newer meters do not require calibration)
• the expiration date on the reagent strips is not exceeded
• the strips are compatible with the blood glucose meter

- the drop of blood covers the entire sample area on the strip (some meters display a message or signal if there is not enough blood)
- the blood glucose level is not read until the test is complete
- there is no major change in temperature, hematocrit, motion, or humidity, as this can affect some blood glucose monitors.

Most blood glucose meters require less than 1 to 2 microliters of blood and give a result in less than 10 seconds. Meters have memories to save past readings that are compatible with computer software programs for comparing long-term blood glucose values to determine effectiveness of blood glucose control. Table 2.1 compares features of some of popular meters.

Products
The following manufacturers make several models of glucose monitors: Abbott, Bayer, Lifescan, and Roche Diagnostics.

Hemoglobin A1c monitors

Blood glucose monitors provide an immediate measure of glucose levels for an individual so that insulin dosage can be adjusted. A better measurement of long-term glucose control is glycoslated hemoglobin (HbA1c). Glucose enters the red blood cell where it combines with hemoglobin and remains there for the lifespan of the red blood cell, 120 days. Values for HbA1c of 7 or less indicate good glucose control and minimize the risks of detrimental health consequences associated with diabetes.

Return mail tests

Mode of action
A drop of blood from a finger stick is placed on a reagent pad on a card and is sent to the manufacturer for analysis. The kit contains lancet, band-aid, reagent card with code number, and return mailer. Several days later, the individual calls the manufacturer on a toll free number and provides the code to a trained counselor who discusses the test's result with the individual.

Product
Appraise Diabetes A1c Test, Reli On A1c Test.

At home test

Mode of action
A drop of blood from a finger stick is placed on a test strip containing reagent. The test strip is inserted into a photoreflectance meter and the result is digitally displayed.

Table 2.1 Selected characteristics of popular blood glucose monitors

Meter	Calibration code	Blood (microliters)	Alternative site testing	Special feature
Abbott				
Free Style Lite	Yes	0.3	Yes	Blood may be added to either side of test strip
Free Style Freedom	Yes	0.3	Yes	
Precision Xtra	Automatic code chip	0.6	Yes	Measures blood glucose and blood ketones; two different strips
Bayer Ascencia				
Breeze 2	No	1.0	Yes	Contains 10 strips loaded in the meter
Contour	No	0.6	Yes	Easy to use
Lifescan One Touch				
Ultra mini	Yes	1.0	Yes	Smallest meter
Ultra	Yes	1.0	Yes	
Ultra Smart	Yes	'Speck'	Yes; finger preferred	Gives averages and graphs results on meter itself; does not need separate computer
Pfizer Accu-Chek				
Compact Plus	No	1.5	Yes	Contains lancet and preloaded 17 strip drum
Aviva	Yes	0.6	Yes	Use wide-mouth strips
Rite Aid				
True Track Smart	No	1.0	Yes	Disposable after the 50 test strips in kit are used

Products
A1cNow, A1c At-Home.

Fecal occult blood in the stool

Individuals who suddenly have very dark or black-looking bowel movements may be experiencing blood loss from the gastrointestinal (GI) tract. A positive result from an OTC fecal occult blood test cannot identify the cause of the bleeding, just its presence. There are many possible causes of fecal blood loss including many common conditions such as peptic ulcer disease, colon cancer, ulcerative colitis, diverticulitis, fissures, and hemorrhoids. Many individuals consider this test to be a cancer screening test, but it is not. Individuals who have a positive test must contact their physician for a proper diagnosis.

Occult blood toilet bowl test

Mode of action
An individual drops a paper impregnated with a dye, tetramethylbenzidine, into the toilet bowl after a bowel movement. The heme (iron) portion of hemoglobin acts as an oxidizing agent, causing a blue-green color on the paper if blood is present. Three successive bowel movements are tested and the result from each is recorded by the individual. If the result is positive on any part of the paper during any one of the three tests, the individual is directed to contact a physician.

Warnings and precautions
Women should avoid testing during menstruation. Irritating substances that may cause GI bleeding should be avoided immediately before and during the testing period. These substances include alcohol, aspirin, caffeine, ibuprofen, naproxen sodium, and any prescription drugs that are gastric irritants. Use of these substances during testing may produce false positive test results.

Products
EZ Detect, First Check Colorectal Test.

Antibody occult blood test

Mode of action
The antibody occult blood test uses the antibody–antigen reaction to detect hemoglobin in a stool sample. A sample of feces is removed from the toilet bowel using a collection stick provided in the kit. The stick is placed in a bottle containing a buffer solution and shaken. Two drops of solution are placed in a test cassette, and after 5 minutes the result is available. A positive result requires consultation with a physician.[5]

Warnings and precautions
Women should avoid testing during menstruation. Irritating substances that may cause GI bleeding should be avoided immediately before and during the testing period. These substances include alcohol, aspirin, caffeine, ibuprofen, naproxen sodium, and any prescription drugs that are gastric irritants.

Product
ColonCARE.

Fertility test kits

When conception is desired, several methods may be used to predict when a mature ovum will be released into the fallopian tubes. Intercourse during this time increases the probability of fertilization of a mature ovum by sperm. These tests include use of monoclonal antibodies to detect hormones, measurement of the body's basal temperature, or monitoring of saliva for electrolyte changes.

The morning's first urine stream usually has the highest level of hormones being tested and provides the best time for measurement when this type of test is being used. Low sperm counts and failure to produce a mature ovum are among the many possible causes of infertility. A physician should be consulted if conception does not occur.

Women taking hormones or fertility drugs should not use these test devices because of possible false results. Certain medical conditions will also produce false results.

Ovulation tests

Monoclonal antibody tests

Mode of action
The pituitary gland releases a high concentration of luteinizing hormone (LH) immediately before ovulation, LH surges. It stimulates the release of a mature ovum into the fallopian tube. The excreted LH can be detected in the urine as soon as this begins using an antibody–antigen reaction.

Since the exact day of the start of the LH surge is not known, the woman must know the length of her menstrual cycle. Ovulation occurs 14 days prior to menstruation and the woman should begin testing for LH a few days before ovulation is expected to begin. A device with a stick at one end containing monoclonal antibody is placed in the morning's first urine stream. The sample moves by capillary attraction to produce a color, a plus sign (+), or some other symbol on the device to indicate the presence of LH, a positive result. A sample of morning's first urine could be collected in a cup and the device placed into the sample cup to do the test instead of using the urine stream.

Ovulation test kits contain multiple test sticks (five to nine sticks) because several days of testing may be necessary to determine when the LH surge begins. The cost of most kits is approximately $30.

Warnings and precautions
Some prescription drugs and medical conditions may produce false positive results.

Products
Clear Blue Easy Ovulation Test, First Response Ovulation Test, Answer Quick and Simple One Step Test, Early Detect Ovulation Test, Accu-Clear Early Ovulation Test.

Luteinizing hormone and estrogen hormone devices

Estrogen levels increase during the follicular stage of the menstrual cycle and peak just before the LH surge occurs. Estrone 3-glucuronide, a metabolite of estrogen, increases in the urine. The detection of both of these hormones may increase the ability of the couple to predict ovulation more accurately.

Mode of action
The test uses antibody–antigen technology to detect LH and estrone 3-glucuronide. A test stick in placed in the stream of the morning's first urine daily beginning on day five in the menstrual cycle and then inserted into the monitor. The monitor displays one of three readings digitally: low, high, or peak fertility.

Warnings and precautions
The woman's menstrual cycle should be between 21 and 42 days. If the woman used birth control pills or was breast feeding, testing should not begin until there have been two normal menstrual cycles. Menopause, liver or kidney disease, polycystic ovarian syndrome, and use of tetracycline may give inaccurate results.[6]

Product
Clear Blue Easy Fertility Monitor. The initial cost of this device is $170 and replacement reagent sticks cost approximately $44 for 30 sticks.

Basal temperature devices

Mode of action
Approximately 24 hours after the LH surge and before ovulation occurs, there is a slight decrease in the body's basal temperature that is followed by a slight increase for a few days, which ranges approximately from 0.5 to 1.0 degrees Fahrenheit (°F) (0.9–1.8°C).

This method is less accurate in predicting ovulation than the antibody–antigen devices but is less costly. A digital thermometer that reads temperature with 0.01°F differences is the only device needed. The woman measures and records her basal body temperature at the same time daily, usually in the morning before getting out of bed. Devices are available with memories and some can be used with computer software packages that allow comparison of temperature changes over multiple menstrual cycles.

Warnings and precautions
Measurements should be after a restful sleep and must be made using the same method. The temperature must be taken before the woman engages any physical activity, like getting out of bed.

Products
Becton Dickinson Basal Thermometer; OvuQuick Basal Thermometer.

Electrolyte test devices

When estrogen levels increase during the menstrual cycle, there is a change in concentration of sodium, potassium, and chloride in saliva and vaginal secretions; this changes the viscosity of these secretions.

Saliva test devices

Mode of action
A sample of saliva from under the tongue is allowed to dry on a glass slide that is viewed daily with a magnifying device provided in the kit. The pattern of dried crystals changes from that of a series of dots or blobs to one that looks like a branched fern.[7]

Product
Fertile-Focus.

Mode of action
The test kit contains a device that is placed on the tongue. It uses an electro-chemical reaction to determine sodium and potassium levels to indicate probability of ovulation.[8]

Product
OvaCue.

Skin test devices

Mode of action
A watch-like device contains a biosensor pad that responds to chloride levels on the skin. It is worn nightly for at least 6 hours approximately 4–5 days before ovulation is expected. Chloride levels increase just before estrogen levels peak during the menstrual cycle, providing another indication that ovulation will occur.[9]

Product
OV-Watch.

Male fertility tests

Sperm Count

Men who have low sperm counts or sperm with impaired motility may not be able to impregnate their partners. Men are often reluctant to see a physician and the use of an OTC home test to determine sperm counts may be helpful in determining a possible cause for infertility.

Mode of action
Ejaculated semen is placed in a collection cup that alters the viscosity of the semen for at least 15 minutes before performing the test. A sample of semen and a control sample are placed in a cassette device. A blue dye is added to the sample and control. If the color of the semen sample is the same as the control sample or darker, the sperm count is at least 20 million per milliliter, a normal value. A color that is less intense than the control indicates a sperm count that is lower than normal. A physician should be consulted if a low sperm count is indicated.[10]

Warnings and precautions
This multistep test may lead to errors during the procedure and produce invalid results. The directions must be followed exactly. If the couple cannot conceive a child, both should consult a physician even if the sperm count is normal.

Products
FertilMARQ, PreConceive Plus Male Fertility Test.

Sperm count and sperm motility

Mode of action
The kit contains a microscope with a grid on the lens. A sample of semen is placed on a slide and viewed through the microscope. Directions provide information of interpreting the view of sperm on the grid and how to compare it with a control sample to determine sperm count and motility.[11]

Product
Micra.

Pregnancy test devices

Human chorionic gonadotropin (hCG) is produced by trophoblastic cells in the corpus luteum within 8 to 10 days after conception and appears in the urine. A morning's first urine sample should contain the highest concentration of hCG and provide the most accurate result. The secretion of hCG increases and peaks at approximately 6 to 8 weeks after fertilization, but then decreases. Performing the test too soon or too late may give an erroneous result.

Mode of action
This test is based on an antibody–antigen reaction. Most test devices will detect hCG levels the first day after a missed menstrual cycle; some devices may detect hCG as early as 5 days after fertilization. A stick impregnated with reagents is placed in the urine stream or in a cup containing a urine sample. Capillary attraction of the urine sample over the reaction area produces a color, plus sign (+), or digital readout to indicate a positive or negative test.

Warnings and precautions
If the concentration of hCG is too low for detection when the test is first done, a negative result will be obtained. The test should be repeated within a week if the possibility of pregnancy exists. Women should consult with their physician if a positive test is obtained. There are some disease states that may produce a false positive result.

Products
Test stick devices include Answer Pregnancy Test, First Response Early Result, Clearblue Easy Earliest Result, e.p.t., Fact Plus, and AccuClear.

Infectious disease kits

Individuals who have unprotected sex or are intravenous drug users who do not use sterile syringes are at high risk for acquiring hepatitis, HIV, and other infections transmitted by biological fluids. Home tests are available for those individuals who suspect that they may have been exposed to these agents. There are no FDA approved home test kits for hepatitis A or hepatitis B at this time.

Hepatitis C

Mode of action
A sample of capillary blood obtained from a finger stick is placed on a reagent pad on a card. The card is closed and sealed and returned to the manufacturer for analysis. After a specified period of time, the individual calls a toll free number, provides the code number from the test, and is given the result of the test. A trained counselor responds to the telephone call and provides additional information to the individual regarding the meaning of the test result and procedures that the individual should follow if the test result is positive.

The test kit contains directions, a lancet, antiseptic pad, band-aid, specimen card with a code number, and a return mailer.

Product
Home Access Hepatitis C Check Kit.

HIV-1

Mode of action
The HIV-1 test is an antibody–antigen test. A sample of capillary blood obtained from a finger stick is placed on a reagent pad on a card. The card is closed and sealed and returned to the manufacturer for laboratory analysis. After a specified period of time, the individual calls a toll free number, provides the code number from the test, and is given the result of the test. A trained counselor responds to the telephone call and provides additional information to the individual regarding the meaning of the test result and procedures that the individual should follow if the test result is positive.

The test kit contains directions, a lancet, antiseptic pad, band-aid, specimen card with a code number, and a return mailer.

Product
Home Access HIV-1 test kit.

Vaginal pH tests

The normal pH of the vagina is acidic, usually around 3.5 to 4.5. If a woman has a vaginal infection caused by bacteria, the vaginal pH usually increases. Women who experience vaginal itching and/or vaginal discharge may have either a bacterial or a fungal/yeast (candida) infection. If the woman had a previous vaginal infection that was diagnosed as a candida infection by a physician, she may purchase an OTC product to treat subsequent infections. OTC vaginal antifungal products are not effective against vaginal bacterial infections.

Often a woman may be in doubt as to whether or not she has a candida infection, and she should consult a physician. However, some women are reluctant to see a physician, and an OTC test that measures vaginal pH may help to distinguish between the two types of infection for these individuals.

Mode of action
Reagents on a test device will change color depending on the pH of the specimen placed on the device. A sample of the vaginal secretion is obtained and the color of the test device is compared with a color guide, indicating the pH of vaginal secretions.

Warnings and precautions
This test is intended for women who have a normal menstrual cycle, because pH is dependent on a number of factors including normal hormone levels. The test should not be performed during menses. Women who are pregnant or

have recently given birth should not use this test. Postmenopausal women should not use this test because low estrogen levels may increase vaginal pH in the absence of a bacterial infection.

The reagent area on the test device should not be touched and may be used only once. If the test is positive, the vaginal pH is higher than normal and the woman should consult a physician. If a negative result is obtained but the woman has symptoms of vaginal itching and discharge, a physician should be consulted regardless of the negative result.

Product

FEM-V. This test consists of a pantiliner that has an insert with reagent on it. The woman uses the pantiliner and the vaginal secretions will wet the insert and react with the reagent. The insert is removed from the pantiliner, placed in a plastic tray and allowed to dry. If a blue–green color appears after 10 minutes, the pH is increased, indicating that a bacterial infection is probably present. This is a positive test and requires proper diagnosis and treatment by a physician. If a yellow color appears after 10 minutes, a candida infection is probably present, and the woman could begin self-care with an OTC product or she could see a physician for a proper diagnosis.[12] *Vagisil Screening Kit.* This kit contains a hand-held device with a circle containing pH paper. It is inserted into the vagina and the paper circle is pressed against the vaginal wall for 5 seconds and removed. The color is matched to a test chart, indicating the pH.[13]

Urinary tract infections

Urinary frequency and urgency and/or discomfort during urination may indicate the presence of a urinary-tract infection. If any blood appears in the urine, a physician must be consulted because self-care is not appropriate even if there are no other symptoms.

Urinary nitrate tests

Mode of action
The bacteria responsible for most urinary-tract infections convert urinary nitrate compounds to nitrites. A test stick containing a reagent is placed in a sample of a morning's first urine stream for 10 seconds. The color produced on the reagent pad is matched with a color chart provided with the kit to determine if the test result is positive.[14]

A positive test result, or a negative test result when the individual has urinary-tract symptoms, requires consultation with a physician.

Products
UTI Home Screening Test Strips, Azo Test Strips.

Urinary nitrates and urinary protein test

Mode of action
Protein (albumin) in the urine may also indicate the presence of an infection. The device contains a stick at one end that is placed in the urine stream. Capillary attraction moves the urine sample to areas on the stick that have reagents to indicate the nitrate to nitrite result in one window on the device and the presence of protein in another window. If either or both tests are positive, the individual should consult a physician. If the individual has urinary-tract symptoms and both tests are negative, the individual should consult a physician. The presence of protein in the urine but not nitrites could indicate the presence of kidney disease.[14]

Product
UTI Bladder Infection Test.

Drugs of abuse screening tests

Urine drug test kits

The FDA approves home test kits that use urine samples to determine the presence of some prescription and illicit drugs. These tests do not provide information about the amount of drug present, just whether or not the drug is present. Prescription drugs in the following pharmacological classes can be detected: barbiturates, benzodiazepines, methadone, opiates (codeine and morphine, and oxycodone), and tricyclic antidepressants. Illicit substances include amphetamine, methamphetamine, cocaine (crack), ecstasy (3,4-methylenedioxymethamphetamine, also known as MDMA), heroin, marijuana (pot), and phencyclidine (PCP or angel dust).[15] Table 2.2 provides information as to how soon after using the drug it may be detected in the urine and how long after use it can be detected.

Mode of action
The drug testing kits contain a urine collection cup with one or more strips, each containing a reagent pad that is viewed for its result. If there is a positive test result, the urine sample may be returned to the manufacturer to confirm the test and determine the amount of drug present. Kits have a code number and the individual either calls a toll free telephone number or goes to a manufacturer's website to obtain the results of laboratory tests.

Products
First Check: First Check 12 drug tests, First Check Marijuana Test, First Check Cocaine Test.

Table 2.2 Drugs that are detected in home tests using urine samples		
Drug	Time for drug to appear in urine after use (h)	Time drug is detectable after ingestion (days)
Marijuana	1–3	1–7
Crack (cocaine)	2–6	2–3
Opiates (heroin)	2–6	1–3
Amphetamines	4–6	2–3
Phencyclidine (PCP or angel dust)	4–6	2–4
Ecstasy	2–7	2–4
Benzodiazepines	2–7	1–4
Barbiturates	2–4	1–3
Methadone	3–8	1–3
Tricyclic antidepressants	8–12	2–7
Oxycodone	1–3	1–2

At Home: At Home 12 drug tests; At Home 5 Drug test kit (marijuana, amphetamine, methamphetamine, cocaine, opiates), At Home Single Test (marijuana), At Home Single Test (cocaine).

Hair follicle test kits

Most drugs are detectable in urine samples for 1 to 3 days after the drug enters the body. However, drugs are also deposited in hair follicles and remain there until the hair grows out and is cut. A hair sample directly from the scalp may contain traces of drugs used as much as 3 months earlier. These test kits have code numbers and the hair sample is returned to the manufacturer for analysis. The individual calls the toll free number, provides the code number, and is told the test's result.[16]

Mode of action
Hair samples are analyzed using gas chromatography and mass spectrometry.

Products
PDT-90, HairConfirm.

Alcohol test kits

Mode of action
An enzyme-based reaction of either a breath sample or a saliva sample converts the alcohol in the sample to a blood alcohol level.

Warnings and precautions

No food or drink should be ingested nor should the individual smoke for at minimum of 10 minutes before the test is performed.[17]

Products

Breath tests: AlcoHAWK Elite Breath Detector; Bactrack Breathalyzer and Safe Drive Deluxe Detector.
Saliva test: Early Detect Blood Alcohol.

Thermometers

Fever thermometers are probably the most frequently purchased devices for home use. Cost for these devices varies widely. Most electronic digital thermometers cost $4.00–10.00; infrared ear thermometers cost $40.00, and infrared temporal artery devices $50.00.

Oral, rectal, and underarm electronic thermometers

A rise in the normal body temperature is often associated with an infection or some other medical condition. Although most people consider the normal body temperature to be 98.6°F (37°C) an individual's temperature may be as much as one degree Fahrenheit higher or lower. The body temperature also varies by approximately 1°F throughout the day. The lowest body temperature occurs just after awakening in the morning and increases to a maximum level in the evening. Increased physical activity also causes an increase in body temperature.

A persistent increase in body temperature indicates that a fever is present. An oral temperature above 100°F (37.8°C) is considered a fever in adults, and a rectal temperature over 100.4°F (38.0°C) is considered a fever in young children. Rectal temperatures are preferred in young children because of their inability to use an oral thermometer correctly. Rectal temperatures may also be used if an individual is unconscious or not able to follow instructions for an oral measurement.

Temperatures taken rectally are generally 1°F (1.8C) higher than temperatures taken orally. However, rectal temperatures must be taken carefully in order to avoid damaging the rectal mucosa. Rectal thermometers should be coated with a lubricant before insertion. Taking a temperature rectally is not esthetically acceptable to many people and other methods for taking temperatures have been developed.

Temperatures taken under the arm (axillary temperature) are used in newborns and infants. This method is less reliable as the child gets older. The thermometer must be placed in the axilla and the arm held against the body for an accurate measurement. The measurements are approximately the same as rectal measurements in infants less than 1 month old but may read as much as 0.5°F or 1°F (0.9–1.8°C) less when used in older infants or children.[18]

Electronic thermometers that have digital readouts reduce errors in measuring body temperatures. Mercury thermometers are no longer sold because of the environmental hazard associated with mercury, but many people may still have mercury thermometers in their homes. These thermometers are safe unless they are broken. The local health department should be consulted for disposal of mercury-containing products.

Mode of action
Electronic thermometers provide reliable measurements in less than a minute and the values are displayed digitally. Some devices require batteries but disposable thermometers are also available.

Products
BD Musical SpongeBob Digital Thermometer, Vicks Comfortflex Thermometer, Vicks Underarm Thermometer, HoMedics Underarm.

Tympanic membrane thermometers

Mode of action
The device is placed in the ear in such a manner that an infrared wave generated by pressing a button strikes the tympanic membrane. The signal returns to the device, which is calibrated and displays the temperature digitally. The device must be held at the correct angle for the device to work properly, and this is more difficult in young children than in older children and adults. Tympanic membrane thermometers usually give readings that are 0.5–1°F (0.9–1.8°C) higher than an oral measurement.[18]

Products
Thermoscan, Omron Ear Thermometer, Vicks Ear Thermometer.

Temporal artery forehead thermometers

Mode of action
The device is drawn across the forehead from its midline to the hair line while an infrared sensor measures heat from the temporal artery. It may be more accurate for infants than tympanic membrane devices. It generally gives a reading that is 1°F (1.8°C) higher than oral body temperatures.[19]

Warnings and precautions
The device should be kept at room temperatures for 30 minutes before using; it should not be used on scar tissue or injured skin; it should not be used outside or if sweat is present of the forehead. Temperature may also be measured over the temporal artery behind the ear at about the level of the ear lobe.[19]

Product
Exergen TAT-2000C.

Ear examination kits

Ear infections are frequent in children and are a leading cause of visits to pediatricians. These devices are intended to help caregivers to determine whether or not a physician should be consulted.

Visual examination of the inner ear

Mode of action
An ear examination kit consists of a user's manual that has pictures of conditions that may affect the middle ear and the tympanic membrane and a medical quality device to see the inner ear. The device is similar to a medical otoscope. The caregiver compares what is seen with photographs in the manual. The pediatrician is called and the caregiver reports what was seen when looking into the inner ear. The physician then provides the caregiver with directions for care of the child.

Product
Dr. Dedo's Ear Examination Kit.

Determination of fluid in the inner ear

Mode of action
Fluid frequently accumulates in the inner ear, which may result in ear pain. A device that generates a sound wave (chirping) is inserted into the outer ear and the signal is reflected from the tympanic membrane to the device. The sound is converted by a microprocessor that indicates whether or not fluid has accumulated. If the test indicates that it is likely that there is fluid present, the caregiver should contact the child's physician.[20]

Warnings and precautions
This device should not be used in children under 6 months of age, in children who have tubes in their ears, in children with perforated ear drum or ear deformities, or if there is any drainage from the ear.[20]

Product
EarCheck Middle Ear Monitor.

Throat examination kits

Mode of action
This kit consists of a user's manual, tongue depressor, and a penlight. The manual contains photographs of the normal throat tissues and various

conditions that may occur in the throat. The caregiver compares the conditions appearing in the throat with the photographs. The pediatrician is called and the caregiver reports what was seen when looking into the throat. The physician instructs the caregiver on the appropriate actions to follow.

Product
Dr. Dedo's Throat Examination Kit.

Breast self-examination kit

Mode of action
A soft plastic, ultra-thin pad contains a lubricant inside to increase tactile sensitivity to an abnormal mass in the breast. The pad is placed over the breast and self-examination of the breast is performed. If any abnormality is detected, a physician should be consulted.

Product
Sensability.

Menopause detection kit

Estrogen levels in women are controlled by the secretion of a hormone from the posterior pituitary gland, follicle stimulating hormone (FSH). When estrogen blood levels fall, FSH is secreted to initiate synthesis of estrogen to return circulating levels to the normal values. Once estrogen levels reach the normal value, the pituitary gland stops secreting FSH.

As a woman approaches menopause, normal production of estrogen decreases, causing the pituitary to continue secreting FSH. Since it is not possible for more estrogen to be synthesized, the levels of FSH continue to be higher than normal.[21]

Mode of action
An antibody–antigen reaction detects the amount of FSH present in the urine. A stick containing monoclonal antibodies is placed in the urine stream. The sample moves along the stick, where the antibody–antigen reaction occurs and produces a positive or negative result. If the test is positive, the woman is advised to consult a physician.

Products
Menocheck, Early Detect Menopause Test Kit, Sure Step FSH Menopause.

Paternity testing

Mode of action
A male who wishes to verify if he is the biological father of a child may submit a biological sample from himself and the child. The samples are sent to the

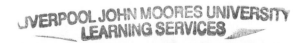

manufacturer and a DNA test is performed using the polymerase chain reaction. The individual calls the toll free number after a specified period of time for the test results.

Product
Paternity Test Kit.

Case study exercises

Case 1 A 48-year-old woman who has a hearing problem asks the pharmacist to recommend a blood pressure monitor because she doesn't know the difference between an aneroid monitor and an electronic monitor.

The pharmacist recommends that she purchase an electronic blood pressure monitor. The aneroid monitor requires that she use a stethoscope to hear the sounds needed for measurement of her blood pressure. Her hearing difficulty may interfere with her ability to hear those sounds. The electronic monitor has sensors in the blood pressure cuff that automatically detects these sounds for measurement.

Case 2 A man asks the pharmacist to recommend a product that he can use to check his cholesterol levels because he takes prescription drugs to lower his triglycerides.

The pharmacist recommends that he consider purchasing CardioChek. This device is able to measure total cholesterol, high-density lipoprotein cholesterol and triglycerides using a small finger stick sample of blood on a reagent strip. He can also calculate his low-density lipoprotein cholesterol. Although he only wants a triglyceride measurement, no home diagnostic tests are available for measuring only triglycerides.

Case 3 A patient who has diabetes wants to measure her hemoglobin A1c and her blood glucose levels. She wants to know if there is a monitor that does both.

The pharmacist tells the woman that there is no single product that can do both; she will have to purchase each device separately.

Case 4 A 52-year-old man asks the pharmacist where the colon cancer test kits are in the pharmacy. His mother had colon cancer and he wants to do a home test because he is afraid to visit a doctor.

The pharmacist advises him that he made an excellent decision to want to be tested for colon cancer because of his family history. However, the home test kits only detect occult blood in the feces. Unfortunately, this test is not specific for colon cancer. Many individuals who have colon cancer may not have any rectally bleeding. The pharmacist strongly recommends that he consult a doctor because of the potential serious nature of his situation.

Case 5 A young woman asks the pharmacist to recommend a product that will improve the chances of getting pregnant as she and her husband have been trying to conceive a child for nearly 18 months and have been unsuccessful; they do not want to see a physician because their health insurance will not cover this type of expense.

The pharmacist suggests she consider purchasing the Clear Blue Easy Fertility Monitor. Although this product is more expensive than most of the other ovulation detecting devices, it measures both luteinizing hormone and estrogen levels, which are used to detect ovulation.

The pharmacist also suggests they consider using an OTC diagnostic test kit to determine whether or not her husband has a sufficient number of sperm with appropriate motility. Several products are available for this purpose.

Case 6 The mother of a 14-year-old child is concerned that the child maybe using drugs and asks the pharmacist to recommend a test product.

The pharmacist explains that she needs to have a discussion with the child about this situation before resorting to a testing procedure. The pharmacist explains that the at-home test kits require a urine sample from the child. There are kits that are specific for certain drugs like marijuana or cocaine or kits that detect drug use without identifying the specific drug. Some test kits require the urine sample be sent to the manufacturer for analysis. There is also a test kit that uses a hair sample for analysis. The hair sample must be cut from near the scalp and returned to the manufacturer for analysis.

Case 7 A 34-year-old woman asks the pharmacist if there is a home test for detecting menopause as her menstrual cycles have been irregular and she gets some hot flashes occasionally, but she thinks she is too young to be entering menopause and she can't afford to go to the doctor.

The pharmacist recommends that she consider purchasing either Menocheck or Sure Step FSH Menopause test. Both of these products determine the level of follicle-stimulating hormone present in the urine. A high level of this hormone indicates that menopause may be occurring, but the woman should consult a physician about her situation.

Case 8 The father of child tells the pharmacist that his wife told him to buy a thermometer that is used in the ear; he says he doesn't know what to buy and he wants the pharmacist to make a recommendation.
The pharmacist explains that there is a device that measures the body temperature by using ultrasound waves that are reflected from the tympanic membrane in the ear. Several manufacturers make these devices including Thermoscan, Omron and Vicks.

References

1. Public Law 94-295, U.S.C. § 321 (h).
2. *FDA Review of Home-Use Devices.* Updated February 1, 2003. www.fda.gov/cdrh/oivd/doc-fdareview.html (accessed December 27, 2008).
3. *Over the Counter Database.* www.accessdata.fda.gov/scripts/cdrh/cfdocs/cfIVD/Search.cfm (accessed December 27, 2008).
4. *Home Test Kits: Cholesterol.* www.fda.gov/cdrh/oivd/homeuse-cholesterol.html (accessed January 24, 2009).
5. ColonCare: Home Use Immunological FOB Test. www.careproductsonline.com/coloncare/index.php (accessed January 24, 2009).
6. Clear Blue Easy Fertility Monitor. www.early-pregnancy-tests.com/clearblue.html (accessed January 24, 2009).
7. Fertile-Focus. www.fertilefocus.com/ (accessed January 24, 2009).
8. OvaCue Fertility Monitor. www.zetek.net/ (accessed January 24, 2009).
9. Ov-Watch Fertility Predictor. www.ovwatch.com/ (accessed January 24, 2009).
10. Baby Start (Fertil MARKQ). www.testsymptomsathome.com/emb01.asp (accessed January 24, 2009).
11. Micra. www.early-pregnancy-tests.com/spermtest.html (accessed January 24, 2009).
12. *Fem-V.* www.biospace.com/news_story.aspx?NewsEntityId=59884 (accessed January 24, 2009).
13. Vagisil. www.vagisil.com/productinformation.shtml (accessed January 24, 2009).
14. *UTI Home Screening Test Strip.* www.utihometest.com/?OVRAW=uti&OVKEY=uti&OVMTC=standard&OVADID=33566545512&OVKWID=12424559012 (accessed January 24, 2009).
15. *Home-use Tests: Drugs of Abuse (First Check 12 Drug Test).* Updates March 3, 2006. www.fda.gov/cdrh/oivd/homeuse-drug-firstcheck 12.html (accessed January 12, 2009).
16. PDT-90 and Hair Confirm. www.testcountry.com/details.html?cat=123 (accessed January 27, 2009).
17. Alcohol tests. www.drugstore.com/search/search_results.asp?N=0&Ntx=mode%2Bmatchallpartial&Ntk=All&srchtree=1&Ntt=alcohol+tests&Go.x=12&Go.y=15 (accessed January 27, 2009).
18. Body temperature. http://firstaid.webmd.com/body-temperature (accessed January 31, 2009).
19. Exergen. www.exergen.com/medical/TAT/2000c.htm (accessed January 31. 2009).
20. EarCheck. http://healthtestingathome.com/earcheckmiddleearmonitorec-2.aspx (accessed January 31, 2009).
21. Menocheck. www.menocheck.com/pages/menochecknews.htm (accessed January 31, 2009).

3

Gastrointestinal system

The process of digestion begins when food enters the mouth and is chewed and mixed with saliva from the salivary glands; this provides lubrication and begins digestion by salivary enzymes. This bolus of food passes through the pharynx and esophagus via the lower esophageal sphincter (LES) into the stomach for further digestion. The LES closes, preventing reflux of the gastric content into the esophagus, where it could cause irritation, and digestion continues in the stomach.

The stomach wall contains cells that secrete acid, mucus, enzymes, and hormones that affect digestion and motility. The bolus enters the small intestine through the pyloric sphincter. Secretions from the intestinal mucosa contain additional enzymes and hormones, affecting motility and enhancing digestion. Secretions from the pancreas, liver, and gall bladder increase fluid volume in the small intestine and further enhance digestion and absorption. Nondigestible materials and metabolic waste products pass into the large intestine for elimination.

Digestive problems affect a large number of people and produce a variety of symptoms, including acid indigestion, upset stomach, sour stomach, heartburn, gastroesophageal reflux disease (GERD), nausea, vomiting, bloating, intestinal gas, constipation, and diarrhea. When these symptoms are mild and occur occasionally, self-care is appropriate. However, these symptoms also occur in individuals who have peptic ulcer diseases, such as gastric ulcers, duodenal ulcers, chronic gastritis, chronic GERD, and hiatus hernia; treatment of these conditions requires supervision by a physician. Many of the OTC drugs in this chapter may be used during treatment of these conditions with prescription medications.

Other symptoms that may occur with the GI symptoms above require immediate referral to a physician, including the presence of blood in the vomit or stools, any difficulty in swallowing or breathing, or the presence of light-headedness, sweating, or pain in the shoulder, arms, neck, or chest. These symptoms indicate a serious condition that cannot be diagnosed by the individual and are not amenable to self-care. Pregnant women and lactating mothers should consult a physician before using any OTC drugs. OTC drugs should not be administered to children 2 years of age or less unless a physician has been consulted.

Acid indigestion, heartburn, GERD, relief of upset stomach associated with overindulgence in food and drink

Antacids

Drug category and indications for use

Antacids provide relief from occasional heartburn, sour stomach, or acid indigestion, and provide relief of upset stomach from food or drink.[1,2]

Monograph ingredients

Aluminum hydroxide, calcium carbonate, magaldrate, magnesium hydroxide, magnesium oxide, sodium bicarbonate, and sodium citrate are the most commonly used ingredients in antacid products.[1] The neutralizing ability varies among these drugs, with sodium bicarbonate, sodium citrate, and calcium carbonate being the more effective neutralizers, followed by magnesium hydroxide and aluminum hydroxide.

All monograph antacids except sodium bicarbonate are approved for symptoms related to upset stomach from overindulgence of food or drink (hangover symptoms), and their use should be limited to 2 days for this purpose. Sodium bicarbonate releases carbon dioxide, and if any undissolved drug is ingested it can react with gastric acid, causing excessive distension of the stomach and possible rupture.[3] The Alka-Seltzer brand of sodium bicarbonate products is very popular, but the product intended for overindulgence use, Alka-Seltzer Wake-Up Call, does not contain any sodium bicarbonate or any antacid; it contains aspirin and caffeine.

Mode of action

Antacids chemically neutralize hydrochloric acid, an irritating substance secreted into the stomach from cells in the gastric mucosa.

Warnings and precautions

No more than the recommended dose should be taken within any 24 hour period, or for more than 2 weeks without the supervision of a physician. If symptoms are severe, occur frequently, or persist for more than 3 months, referral to a physician is appropriate.

If the individual is taking a prescription drug, a physician or pharmacist should be consulted because drug–drug interactions may occur. Many antacids alter absorption of prescription drugs and should be administered 1 hour before or 2 hours after taking prescription drugs.[1,4]

Sodium bicarbonate and sodium citrate antacids exceed 5 milliequivalents (140 mg) of sodium per daily dose and should not be used by individuals on salt-restricted diets. Tablets or powders containing sodium bicarbonate must be added to at least 4 ounce (120 mL) of water and be dissolved before ingestion.[1] There may be some white residue at the bottom of the glass, but this is not sodium bicarbonate and is safe to ingest. These products produce a vigorous effervescence (bubbling) when carbon dioxide gas is produced; this subsides when all the gas has been released.

Aluminum hydroxide has astringent properties and frequently causes constipation. Magnesium compounds are soluble and frequently cause diarrhea. Manufacturers combine aluminum hydroxide and magnesium hydroxide as a mixture in an effort to balance the bowel effects of these two drugs, with modest success. Magaldrate is a chemical compound of both aluminum and magnesium hydroxides that does not have any particular advantage over products that are physical mixtures. Calcium carbonate may cause constipation and is also combined with magnesium antacids.[1]

Individuals with kidney disease should avoid magnesium antacids if they contain more than 50 milliequivalents of magnesium unless under the supervision of a physician.[1]

Recommended doses
Antacids have a short duration of action. They should be administered 1 hour after meals and as frequently as every 2 to 4 hours as needed. Doses vary and depend on the acid-neutralizing capacity of the individual ingredients. Table 3.1 contains dosage recommendations.

Products
Aluminum hydroxide (AlternaGEL), sodium bicarbonate (Alka-Seltzer Regular Strength, Alka-Seltzer Extra Strength, Alka-Seltzer Gold, Bromo-seltzer), sodium citrate (Alka-Seltzer Heartburn Relief), calcium carbonate (Chooz, Children's Mylanta, Pepto-Bismol Children's Chewable Tablets, Rolaids, Tums, TumsEX, Tums Ultra, Tums Kids, Titralac), magaldrate (Riopan), magnesium hydroxide (Milk of Magnesia), aluminum hydroxide and magnesium hydroxide mixtures (Maalox, Mylanta).

Table 3.1 Usual recommended doses for antacids			
Antacid	Over 12 years and adult	6–11 years	2–5 years
Aluminum hydroxide	600–1200 mg	Consult doctor	Consult doctor
Calcium carbonate	500–1000 mg	400–800 mg	400 mg
Magnesium hydroxide/ aluminum hydroxide	400–800 mg of each every 4 h	Consult doctor	Consult doctor
Sodium bicarbonate	2000 mg every 4 h	1000 mg ever 4 h	Consult doctor

Some popular sodium bicarbonate products (Alka-Seltzer Original and Alka-Seltzer Extra Strength) contain aspirin, a gastric irritant that may aggravate an upset stomach and may cause gastric bleeding.

Some aluminum hydroxide and magnesium hydroxides contain alginic acid and/or sodium alginate as a labeled inactive ingredient because neither has any antacid activity. These substances float on top of the gastric contents and block the LES to prevent acid reflux into the esophagus (GERD). Gaviscon is an example of one of these products. Individuals who have GERD should not lie down after eating as this will reduce the risk of developing heartburn symptoms.

Many individuals, especially women, purchase calcium carbonate formulations that have a high calcium carbonate content, such as TumsEX (750 mg) or Tums Ultra (1000 mg), for use as a source of calcium for bone health. Viactiv Calcium Soft Chews contain calcium carbonate but it is marketed as a source of calcium, not as an antacid.

Bismuth subsalicylate

Drug category and indications for use
Bismuth subsalicylate relieves symptoms of upset stomach caused by over-indulgence in food and drink, including heartburn, nausea, fullness, belching, and gas.[5]

Mode of action
Bismuth subsalicylate provides relief primarily by adhering to the mucosa of the stomach and protecting it from direct contact with stomach acid. It has no antacid ability.

Warnings and precautions
Individuals taking anticoagulants (blood thinning drugs) should consult their physicians before use; there may be a temporary darkening of the tongue and stools from use of this drug. Bismuth subsalicylate products do not contain aspirin but could cause an adverse effect in those allergic to aspirin. It should not be used in children or teenagers who have or are recovering from chickenpox or flu-like symptoms (Reye's syndrome warning).[2,5,6]

Reye's syndrome occurs in children and adolescents under 18 years of age after they have recovered from common viral infections. The risk of developing this condition is increased if aspirin and salicylate drugs are used. Although Reye's syndrome in relatively uncommon, it is a concern because it affects the liver and brain and may cause death.

Recommended dose
Adults and children over age 12 may take 2 tablets (525 mg) every 30 to 60 minutes, but should not exceed eight doses within 24 hours; children aged 9 to

12 may take one-half the adult dose (1 tablet (262 mg); children aged 6 to 9 may take two-thirds of the adult dose (175 mg); children aged 3 to 6 may take one-third of the adult dose (88 mg); children under age 3 require recommendation by a physician.[6]

Products
Pepto-Bismol Caplets, Pepto-Bismol Chewable Tablets (Original), Pepto-Bismol Suspension (Original). Names of products must be exact because the manufacturer has similarly named products that have different active ingredients. For example, Pepto-Bismol Children's Chewable Tablets contain the antacid calcium carbonate, while Pepto-Bismol Chewable Tablets (Original) contain bismuth subsalicylate. All product labels for OTC drugs must be read very carefully before choosing a particular product for use. This situation occurs with many manufacturers and many OTC products.

Histamine H_2-receptor blockers or antagonists

All H_2-blockers take longer to relieve symptoms than antacids, but they have a much longer duration of action. H_2-blockers and antacids may be used together.

Drug category and indications for use
The histamine H_2-receptor blockers are used for temporary relief, or prevention of symptoms of heartburn, indigestion, and sour stomach.

Rx–OTC switched drugs
Cimetidine, famotidine, nizatidine, and ranitidine are the H_2-blockers available as OTC drugs. One formulation of famotidine combines it with calcium carbonate and magnesium hydroxide, two antacids, to provide both fast and prolonged relief. H_2-blockers may be taken before or after meals to prevent or treat GI symptoms.

Mode of action
The release of histamine in the body activates receptors, H_2-receptors, on parietal cells in the stomach to secrete a protein tyrosine kinase that activates the enzyme hydrogen/potassium adenosine triphosphatase (H^+/K^+-ATPase). This is an enzyme on the surface of the parietal cells that uses the energy derived from ATP hydrolysis to drive the exchange of ions (hydrogen, chloride, and potassium ions) across the cell membrane. The net result is the release of hydrogen ions into the stomach where they form hydrochloric acid. The H_2-blockers bind to the same receptors on the parietal cells as histamine, preventing activation of these receptors and, ultimately, preventing the formation of hydrochloric acid in the stomach. Since histamine is one of the most potent stimulators of gastric acid in the body, H_2-blockers are highly effective drugs in relieving heartburn symptoms.

Table 3.2 Usual recommended doses for H_2-receptor blocking drugs		
Drug	Dose (mg)	Use
Cimetidine	200	Take with food or up to 30 min before eating; maximum 2 doses per day
Famotidine	10 or 20	Take 15–60 min before eating; maximum 2 doses per day
Nizatidine	75	Take with meals or up to 60 min before meal; maximum 2 doses per day
Ranitidine	75 or 150	Take 30–60 min before eating; maximum 2 doses per day

Warnings and precautions

These drugs should not be taken for longer than 2 weeks or given to children under 12 years of age. A physician should be consulted if the symptoms persist or are more severe.

Cimetidine inhibits cytochrome P-450 enzymes and patients taking theophylline, phenytoin, or warfarin should consult their physician before using cimetidine.[7] Pharmacists should probably recommend the other H_2-antagonists as a first choice instead of cimetidine because of its P-450 enzyme-inhibiting action.

Recommended dose

Table 3.2 lists the dose for H_2-blockers and their onset of action.

Products

Cimetidine (Tagamet HB), famotidine (Pepcid AC, 10 mg; Pepcid AC Maximum Strength, 20 mg), nizatidine (Axid AR), and ranitidine (Zantac 75 mg and Zantac 150 mg), famotidine and calcium carbonate combination (Pepcid Complete and Tums Dual Action).

Proton pump inhibitors

Drug category and indications for use

Proton pump inhibiting drugs (PPIs) are used for frequent heartburn, which is defined as heartburn that occurs two or more days a week.

Rx–OTC switched drugs

Omeprazole magnesium is the only OTC PPI available on the market at this time; however, the FDA approved the switch of lansoprazole (Prevacid) from Rx–OTC status in May 2009. It will probably be available in the near future.

Mode of action
The PPIs bind irreversibly to the H^+/K^+-ATPase pump in the parietal cell, preventing secretion of acid into the stomach. Because the binding is irreversible, these drugs are the most effective acid reducers and are the preferred drugs when heartburn symptoms are caused by GERD; however, it takes 1 to 4 days for them to achieve their maximum effect. The PPIs and H_2-blockers should not be taken together because both categories act by suppressing acid secretion. Antacids may be used with PPIs.

Warnings and precautions
The PPIs should not be taken for longer than 14 days or if symptoms persist or worsen, without consulting a physician. They should not be used by those under 18 years of age. PPIs may cause diarrhea, headache, abdominal pain, or a rash. Omeprazole magnesium inhibits the P-450 enzymes CYP2C19 and CYP3A4 and should not be used without physician supervision by anyone taking warfarin, diazepam, digoxin, ketoconazole, or itraconazole.[8]

Recommended dose
Omeprazole, 20 mg, should be taken daily with a glass of water for 14 consecutive days, 15 to 60 minutes before eating breakfast or the first meal of the day. Omeprazole begins to produce its effect when parietal cells begin to secrete hydrogen ions under stimulation by food; therefore, it is most effective when taken before eating. This dosage regimen may be repeated once after 4 months if needed. If symptoms are not relieved after a second trial of 14 days of treatment, a physician should be consulted.

The FDA is currently considering an Rx–OTC switch of the prescription drug Zegerid. Zegerid combines omeprazole with sodium bicarbonate to provide rapid heartburn relief from the antacid until the slower-acting omeprazole reaches effective concentrations to produce a prolonged effect.

Product
Omeprazole magnesium (Prilosec OTC).

Gas and bloating

Antiflatulents

Drug category and indications for use
Antiflatulents are intended to relieve symptoms of gas, which include the sensation of abdominal distention, pressure, bloating, feeling of fullness, and belching. Swallowing of air during talking, eating or drinking is a frequent cause of gas. Individuals who experience heartburn, acid indigestion, and upset stomach problems complain that these symptoms are accompanied by gas and belching.[1]

Monograph ingredients

Simethicone is the only antiflatulent approved in the FDA's monograph as a single ingredient and as an ingredient that may be combined with antacid formulations.[1]

Infant colic is a relatively common condition characterized by excessive crying, passing of gas, and assumed gastric distress because the infant draws its legs inward to the abdomen. Simethicone has been used together with alterations in the infant's diet to alleviate this condition. Unfortunately, controlled studies have failed to prove the efficacy of simethicone over placebo in treating infant colic. However, simethicone's lack of adverse effects and the lack of any other clear treatment for infant colic are reasons for its continued use in this condition.[9]

Mode of action

Simethicone reduces the surface tension of gas bubbles present in the stomach, causing them to break up into smaller ones that can be expelled from the GI tract more easily. Simethicone has no antacid activity but it is combined with antacids because gas is a frequent symptom that occurs when heartburn is present.[1]

Warnings and precautions

The only warnings for simethicone are not to exceed the recommended dosage on the label in a 24 hour period unless directed to do so by a physician.

Recommended dose

Simethicone should be taken after meals and before bedtime. The dose for infants under 2 years of age, or less than 24 lbs (10.9 kg) is 20 mg, with a maximum of 240 mg daily; for infants over 2 years of age or 24 lbs, the dose is 40 mg with a maximum of 480 mg. The maximum daily dosage for adults and children over 12 years is 500 mg per day, and single dose recommendations range from 80 to 180 mg.[10]

Products

Simethicone (Mylicon Infant Drops, Phazyme Maximum Strength Chewable Tablets and Softgel Capsules, Mylanta Gas Maximum Strength Chewable Tablets and Softgel Capsules, and Gas X Thin Strips, Chewable Tablets and Softgel Capsules).

Alternative therapy

Alpha-galactosidase

Drug category and indications for use

Alpha-galactosidase is an enzyme that the FDA has approved as a food additive dietary supplement to treat bloating and intestinal gas.

Mode of action

Alpha-galactosidase helps to metabolize oligosaccharides, which are large complex carbohydrate molecules that occur in high fiber foods such as beans, to simpler sugar molecules before they reach the large intestine. Complex carbohydrates are metabolized by bacteria present in the large intestine, producing gas.[11]

Warnings and precautions

One product that contains alpha-galactosidase, Beano, contains a small amount of gluten, and individuals who are sensitive to gluten should consult their physician before use.[11]

Recommended dose

Alpha-galactosidase should be taken immediately before meals or with meals containing foods that produce gas symptoms. The amount of enzyme to be taken depends on the amount of food to be eaten, and specific directions are on product labels. Alpha-galactosidase is available as oral tablets or as powder or liquids to be added to foods before eating. Cooking foods with alpha-galactosidase will reduce or destroy its enzyme activity. It is not recommended for use in children under 12 years of age without a physician's supervision.

Products

Alpha-galactosidase (Beano tablets and liquid).

Peppermint oil

Drug category and indications for use

Peppermint oil is an aromatic oil that is a GRASE drug and has been used to treat abdominal fullness and bloating.

Mode of action

Aromatic oils are thought to relax muscles in the GI tract to produce their effect. Recent evidence demonstrated that peppermint oil relaxes muscle of the LES and is thought to reduce tension created in the stomach from any gas that is present. If this is indeed the mode of action of peppermint oil, it may actually worsen symptoms of heartburn and indigestion caused by gastric reflux (GERD). Peppermint oil is used as a flavoring agent in low doses, including in many antacid and antiflatulent suspensions and tablets. Peppermint oil as a flavoring agent probably has very little effect on LES pressure.[12]

Warnings and precautions

When peppermint oil is used in high doses, it may cause nausea, heartburn, and perianal burning.

Recommended dose

Adult doses range from 0.2 to 0.4 mL up to three times a day; doses for children over 8 years of age range from 0.1 to 0.2 mL up to three times a day.

Product

Peppermint oil.

Nausea and vomiting

Nausea and vomiting have many causes, including local irritation of the gastric mucosa, alterations of gastric motility, and stimulation of the brain by several mechanisms. Several neurotransmitters are involved in producing emesis, including acetylcholine, dopamine, and serotonin (5-hydroxytryptamine).

The common causes of nausea and vomiting that are self-diagnosed and self-treated are motion sickness and local irritation from food and drink. Vomiting causes both fluid and electrolyte loss; if it persists for more than 24 to 48 hours, an individual should consult a physician.

Antiemetics for motion sickness

Drug category and indications for use

Antiemetics are drugs that prevent or treat nausea, vomiting and/or dizziness associated with motion sickness. Motion sickness involves stimulation of nerves of the vestibular apparatus (semicircular canals) of the inner ear, which are responsible for maintaining balance and equilibrium. Signals from the vestibular nerves stimulate cholinergic centers in the vomiting center of the medulla of the brain and this activates cranial nerves and causes muscles in the GI tract to expel gastric content. Vertigo causes some symptoms that are similar to motion sickness, but there are other causes of vertigo that require diagnosis by a physician. Only motion sickness is a self-treatable condition.[13]

Motion sickness is usually precipitated by riding in any type of motor vehicle, train, boat, or airplane. Amusements rides, especially those with circular motion, are likely to cause motion sickness.

All of the OTC antiemetics are antihistamines that have anticholinergic activity. These drugs block the action of acetylcholine both centrally in the brain and peripherally in the parasympathetic nervous system.

Monograph ingredients

OTC antiemetics include cyclizine, dimenhydrinate, diphenhydramine, and meclizine.

Warnings and precautions
These antiemetics may cause drowsiness and should not be used with alcohol, sedatives, or tranquilizers. Caution is required if driving a motor vehicle or operating machinery when using these drugs. The degree of drowsiness depends on the specific chemical structure of the drug, dimenhydrinate and diphenhydramine causing the greatest degree of drowsiness. Meclizine causes the least drowsiness and some of its products contain the words 'less drowsy' in their names.[13]

These drugs should not be taken unless directed by a physician by anyone who has breathing problems (such as shortness of breath, emphysema or chronic bronchitis), glaucoma, or difficulty in urination owing to enlargement of the prostate gland.

Recommended dose
Antiemetics should be taken 30 to 60 minutes before engaging in the activity that causes motion sickness. Recommended dosages for these drugs are listed in table 3.3.

Products
Cyclizine (Marezine, Bonine for Kids), dimenhydrinate (Dramamine), diphenhydramine (Benadryl), and meclizine (Bonine, Dramamine Less Drowsy).

Alternative therapy: ginger

Drug category and indications for use
Ginger is a dietary supplement that is a GRAS drug and used to treat nausea and vomiting; it may have some effect in preventing motion sickness. Ginger

Table 3.3 Usual recommended doses for motion sickness drugs

Drug	Age (years)	Dose
Cyclizine	6–12	25 mg, 6–8 h
	Over 12 and adults	50 mg, 4–6 h
Dimenhydrinate	2–6	12.5–25 mg, 6–8 h
	6–12	25–50 mg, 6–8 h
	Over 12 and adults	50–100 mg, 4–6 h
Diphenhydramine	6–12	12.5–25 mg, 4–6 h
	Over 12 and adults	25–50 mg, 4–6 h
Meclizine	Adults only	25–50 mg, once daily

has demonstrated effectiveness for nausea and vomiting associated with pregnancy, but no medications should be recommended for pregnant women without the approval of their physician.

Mode of action
Ginger inhibits serotonin receptors in the GI tract and the brain and may prevent both local and central stimulation of nerves that cause vomiting.[14]

Warnings and precautions
Ginger may cause heartburn, diarrhea, or irritation of the oral mucosa. It may increase the risk of bleeding if an individual is taking warfarin.

Recommended dose
Powered ginger 250–1000 mg up to four times a day.

Product
Ginger powder.

Phosphorylated carbohydrates

Drug category and indications for use
Concentrated carbohydrates may relieve nausea associated with upset stomach or intestinal flu.

Mode of action
Phosphorylated carbohydrates are theorized to alter gastric emptying to provide relief but the actual mode of action is unknown.[13] A common home remedy for nausea is the use of concentrated coke syrup and its use is based on this same theory.

Warnings and precautions
Phosphorylated carbohydrate products contain 1.87 g glucose and fructose (levulose) and 21.5 mg phosphoric acid per 5 mL. Individuals who have diabetes should not use these products without consulting their physicians; individuals who have fructose intolerance should not use these products.[15]

Recommended dose
Children 2 to 12 years of age may take 5 to 10 mL every 15 minutes until symptoms subside, but should not take more than five doses in an hour; adults and children over 12 years of age may take 15 to 30 mL every 15 minutes until symptoms subside, but also should not take more than five doses in an hour. Phosphorylated carbohydrates should not be diluted with liquids before ingestion.[15]

Products
Phosphorylated carbohydrates (Emetrol and Nausetrol).

Devices for preventing or treating nausea

Mechanical devices

Activation of certain pressure points in the body based on Chinese acupuncture and acupressure, P6 or nei-kuan have demonstrated the ability to suppress nausea.[16] The FDA approved two types of device for motion sickness and for nausea associated with pregnancy (morning sickness).

Mode of action
Adjustable wrist bands containing a bead are placed on the underside of both wrists to create acupressure by the bead. The amount of pressure is adjustable and the bands should be used approximately 5 minutes before travel or motion begins.

Products
Sea-Band and Psi Band. These devices cost less than $10.00.

Electronic devices

Mode of action
A battery-powered wrist band provides an electronic pulse to the underside of the wrist to prevent nausea. A conductivity gel must be applied to the wrist before wearing the device. The device is adjusted so that a pulse or tingling feeling is felt in the palm of the hand or in the middle fingers.[17]

Warnings and precautions
The device should not be used if the individual has a cardiac pacemaker. The device also contains latex and should not be used by anyone having a latex allergy. Mild skin irration may occur. If the irritation is not relieved in 24 hours, a physician or pharmacist should be consulted. The device is not waterproof and should not be submerged in water.[17]

Product
Relief Band. This device costs $130.00.

Poison treatment drug products

Ipecac syrup

Accidental oral ingestion of toxic substances has many potentially serious adverse effects, including death. As long as the ingested substance remains in the GI tract, it continues to be absorbed into the blood stream and will be distributed to all body tissues. Emptying the stomach contents as soon as possible, within 60 to 90 minutes at the latest, reduces the amount of toxin available for absorption. Gastric lavage and vomiting are two mechanisms to remove contents from the stomach.

There is considerable debate as to the overall effectiveness of ipecac within the medical community. The FDA held a meeting of its advisory committee in 2003 to discuss continuing its general recommendation for using ipecac syrup in poisoning situations. Discussions also considered continuing the OTC availability of ipecac because of the potential for abuse by individuals who have eating disorders like bulimia. The FDA has not issued any report or recommendations based on this meeting, and its original approval of ipecac syrup continues.

The American Association of Poison Control Centers issued guidelines in 2005 for using ipecac syrup in treating poisoning victims outside hospital settings. Included among those recommendations were that universal recommendations for ipecac use should be avoided except under the following conditions: (1) there are no contraindications to its use; (2) the risk of injury to the individual from the toxin is substantially greater than the risk associated with ipecac syrup use; (3) the individual would not be able to get emergency treatment within an hour; (4) the ipecac syrup could be administered within 90 minutes of ingestion of the toxin; and (5) no alternative treatment is available for the individual. The Association was not in favor of promoting households to maintain a supply of ipecac syrup. They did not take any position regarding keeping ipecac syrup as an OTC or restricting its use.[18]

Drug category and indications for use
Ipecac syrup is intended for emergency use to cause vomiting of swallowed poisons.[18]

Monograph ingredients
Ipecac syrup is approved by the FDA and restricted for sale to 1 ounce containers for OTC use.

Mode of action
Ipecac syrup contains the alkaloids cephaeline and emetine, which cause local irritation of the stomach mucosa and stimulate the vomiting center in the brain via the chemoreceptor zone. Emetine has the potential to cause cardiac and renal toxicity in excess dose or long-term use.

Warnings and precautions
Ipecac syrup or other emetics should never be used in semiconscious or unconscious individuals, nor should they be used in individuals who are uncooperative or who have any blockage of their airway. Vomiting should not be induced in individuals who have ingested caustic or corrosive substance or products containing petroleum distillates, such as kerosene, gasoline, paint thinner, cleaning fluid, furniture polish, or turpentine. Caustics and corrosives, include alkali (lye) and strong acids, produce damage to the mucosa of the mouth, pharynx, and esophagus during swallowing that will be exacerbated during vomiting. Vomiting may result in aspiration of the vomitus

into the lungs and may result in lipid pneumonia if petroleum products are aspirated. Milk should not be taken with ipecac syrup.[19]

Recommended dose
Before administering ipecac syrup, attempts should be made to contact a poison control center, emergency medical facility, or health professional. Infants under 6 months of age should not be given ipecac syrup unless directed by a health professional. Infants aged 6 months to 1 year of age may be given 5 mL of ipecac syrup mixed with 4 to 8 ounces (120–240 mL) of water or clear liquid; children between age 1 and 12 years of age may be given 15 mL of ipecac syrup mixed with 8 to 16 ounces (240–480 mL) of water or clear liquid; children over 12 years of age and adults may be given 30 mL with 8 to 16 ounces (240–480 mL) of water or clear liquid. If individuals do not vomit within 20 minutes, a second dose of ipecac syrup may be administered.[19]

Individuals should not be given activated charcoal until vomiting occurs. Individual should be kept active and moving if possible.

Activated charcoal

Drug category and indications for use
Activated charcoal is used to adsorb swallowed poisons in emergency situations.[19]

Mode of action
Activated charcoal particles possess a very large surface area. Toxins present in the GI tract will adhere to its surface, preventing or reducing their absorption into the blood stream. The drug and adsorbed toxin are eliminated via the feces. Not all toxins are absorbed by activated charcoal.

Warnings and precautions
Activated charcoal should not be given to an individual until vomiting has occurred unless directed by a health professional; it should not be administered to individuals who are not fully conscious or individuals with an intestinal blockage. It should not be used if the individual has ingested turpentine; corrosives, such as alkali (lye); strong acids; petroleum distillates, such as kerosene or gasoline; paint thinner; cleaning fluid; or furniture polish unless directed by a health professional. Individuals should be informed that bowel movements will be black in color.[19]

Recommended dose
Attempts should be made to contact a poison control center, emergency medical facility or health professional before administering activated charcoal. As soon after the toxin is ingested as possible or as directed by a health

professional, 20 to 30 g of powdered activated charcoal is given in a minimum of 8 ounces (230 mL) of water. Activated charcoal remains as a suspension and should be shaken well before use. Some products are flavored suspensions that improve palatability, which may promote greater acceptance by individuals, especially children, to drink the product. Ipecac syrup and activated charcoal should not be used at the same time.[19]

Products
Activated charcoal (ActiDose Aqua, ActiDose with Sorbitol, EZ-Char, Liqui Char and Insta-Char).

Prevention

Some common sense actions can prevent accidental ingestion of drugs and household substances by young children, who are the individuals involved most frequently in accidental poisonings: all medications and household cleaning supplies should be stored out of reach of children (tall or locked cabinets); children's medications, including vitamins, should not be promoted as being like or tasting like candy; the physician's telephone should be posted in a convenient place for emergency use; the local poison control center's telephone number should be posted in the same place, as should the number of the national poison control number, 1–800–222–1222; the container of the product should be in your hand when making telephone calls so that the product's exact name and ingredients can be readily identified; the product should be taken with you to the emergency room once you have found out which hospital in your area is best able to handle your specific problem.

Pinworms

Pryantel pamoate

Drug category and indications for use
An OTC anthelmintic drug is used to treat infestation by pinworms (*Enterobiasis vermicularis*). No other worm infestation is amenable to OTC treatment.[20]

Pinworms inhabit the small and large intestine after oral ingestion of the larvae. The larvae mature and remain in the intestine for their lifetime. The female pinworm migrates down the intestinal tract during the night and deposits her eggs in the large intestine and around the anal sphincter. This causes intense nocturnal anal itching, the characteristic symptom associated with this condition. Female pinworms are approximately 0.25 to 0.5 inches (0.63–1.25 cm) in length and can be seen at the anal sphincter area during the night. They may also be present in the stools and appear as white, threadlike contaminants.

Scratching because of the intense itching contaminates fingers and hands and can be a source of re-entry into the body if hand and fingernail beds are not thoroughly cleaned. Larvae may survive for up to 3 weeks in contaminated clothing, bedding, and bath towels, and on other surfaces.

Pinworms usually affect young children and it is not uncommon for an entire family to become infected. Infected individuals should wear tight-fitting underwear to reduce contamination, and clothing and bedding must be washed in hot, soapy water. Items that are handled by individuals with pinworms must be disinfected, especially areas in the bathroom such as the toilet seat, tub or shower, and all faucet and door handles.

Mode of action

Pyrantel pamoate acts as a depolarizing neuromuscular blocker in the pinworm. It prevents the worm from clinging to the intestinal mucosa to obtain its nutrients and so it dies. There is no need to use laxative products to remove the affected pinworms from the GI tract.[20]

Warnings and precautions

Abdominal cramps, nausea, vomiting, diarrhea, headache, or dizziness may occur after taking pyrantel pamoate, and a physician should be consulted if the condition persists. The drug should not be taken by those with liver disease unless directed by a physician.[20]

Recommended dose

The dose for adults and children aged 2 years and older is based on the individual's weight and is 11 mg per kilogram (5 mg per pound) body weight. The maximum dose is 1 g. A single oral dose is required, and the entire family should be treated at the same time. If there is a recurrence of pinworms, a second dose should not be taken unless advised to do so by a physician.[20]

Products

Pyrantel pomoate (Reese's Pinworm as capsules or liquid; Pin X as liquid and chewable tablets).

Laxatives

Once digestion and absorption of food are completed, waste products move through the small intestine into the large intestine, where the fecal mass is temporarily stored until defecation occurs. This passage of waste material through the GI tract depends on many factors, but the two most important factors are GI motility and absorption of fluids, primarily water.

Gastric motility is affected by the physical bulk of foods in the diet, the appropriate functioning of the autonomic nervous system, both sympathetic and parasympathetic, hormones, and other substances secreted by the body. If enough bulk, both solid and liquid, is not present in the lumen of the intestines, receptors in the mucosal lining cannot be activated to move the ingested mass along the GI tract.

The sympathetic nervous system controls slow segmental waves for mixing materials that have been ingested, and the parasympathetic nervous system controls peristaltic waves that move the ingested material through the GI tract. The parasympathetic nervous system has a more prominent role in overall GI motility than the sympathetic nervous system.

Hormones and other substances secreted by the body's tissues and organs may increase or decrease motility along the GI tract and may increase or decrease secretions into the GI tract. The major GI hormones include gastrin, which is secreted by the stomach and stimulates gastric acid and enzyme secretions and increases GI motility; secretin, which is secreted by the small intestine and stimulates the pancreas, gall bladder and liver to increase secretions; and cholecystokinin, which is secreted by the small intestine and slows gastric emptying. The intestine also produces gastric inhibitory peptide, which inhibits gastric acid secretion and gastric motility, and motilin, which stimulates intestinal motility.[21]

The normal balance of these substances allows movement through the GI tract at a rate that permits adequate absorption of nutrients, water, and other fluids. Contents from the stomach have a thin, liquid consistency as they enter the small intestine, where secretions from the liver and gall bladder are added to the duodenum, the first portion of the small intestine. As the mass continues through the duodenum into the jejunum and ilium, the other two portions of the small intestine, most nutrients and fluids are absorbed. The mass becomes less liquid as it reaches the large intestine (colon), where excess water is absorbed, and the semisolid feces remains in the colon until evacuation occurs. The daily volume of fluid entering the GI tract is approximately 7000 mL, which is reduced to approximately 100–200 mL of feces ultimately excreted.[21]

A bowel movement (defecation) is achieved by stimulation of stretch receptors in the large intestine and activation of muscles that push the fecal material through the anal sphincter to eliminate the body's solid waste.

The process of digestion, absorption, and elimination of ingested nutrients is a complicated process involving many factors that must be evaluated before deciding the type of laxative appropriate for solving an individual's problem of constipation. The categories of drug used to treat constipation include agents that provide bulk and agents that alter GI motility either directly or indirectly. Table 3.4 describes general characteristics of the different types of laxative.

Any abrupt change in eating habits may be a cause of constipation. Traveling though different time zones changes the time that meals are consumed as well as sleeping patterns, and changing the type of food eaten or the volume of fluids ingested also affects bowel habits. Many prescription and

Table 3.4 Characteristics of laxatives

Laxative category	Approximate onset of action	Effect on electrolyte loss
Bulk formers	2–72 h	Minimal
Lubricants	6–8 h	Minimal
Hyperosmotics or saline laxatives	2–6 h	Maximum
Osmotics (PEG 3350)	12–72 h	Minimal to moderate
Stimulant (irritant or secretory)	6–12 h	Moderate
Stool softeners (docusate)	12–72 h	Minimal
Enemas	2–15 min	Minimal
Suppositories		
Glycerin	15–60 min	Minimal
Carbon dioxide	5–30 min	Minimal
Bisacodyl	15–60 min	Minimal

OTC drugs reduce GI motility, including opioid analgesics, codeine cough suppressants, antihypertensive medications, antihistamines, antidepressants, diuretics, and antacids. Many common medical conditions may cause constipation, including intestinal obstruction, hypothyroidism, diabetes, Parkinson's disease, spinal cord injuries, and multiple sclerosis.

Constipation is a common complaint among the elderly. Several factors may contribute to constipation including an age-related decrease in GI motility, decline in physical activity and a more sedentary lifestyle, and dietary choices.

Any change in normal bowel habits that causes persistent constipation or diarrhea not associated with any of the previous situations warrants a recommendation to a physician for evaluation. Sudden and persistent changes in bowel habits are frequently the first symptoms of colon cancer in many individuals.

Bulk laxatives

Monograph laxatives

Drug category and indications for use

Laxatives are drugs that are intended for the short-term relief, 1 week, of the symptoms of constipation. A common misconception is in the definition of constipation. The FDA monograph definition includes the following:

(1) infrequent bowel movements; (2) difficulty or pain in during defecation; and (3) excessive dry or insufficient quantity of stools. A common misconception is that a bowel movement is required daily. Medically, the frequency may range from three bowel movements a day to three per week. If an individual experiences a sudden change in bowel habit that lasts for 2 weeks or more, a physician should be consulted because this is often a symptom associated with a more serious condition such as obstruction or colon cancer.[22]

Mode of action

Bulk laxatives are replacements for lack of foods containing fiber, such as fruit and vegetables, in an individual's diet. The daily diet should contain approximately 25 to 50 g fiber. The lack of bulk results in failure of activation of receptors necessary for defecation. Dietary bran, guar gum, psyllium (plantago seed), cellulose and methylcellulose, malt soup extract, polycarbophil, and polycarbophil calcium are OTC monograph bulk laxatives.[22]

Psyllium also appears in many food products, especially cereals. Fiber binds fats and lipids from foods, and soluble fiber such as oatmeal is more effective than insoluble fiber like psyllium in this process. This reduction of fat and lipid absorption in the GI tract may reduce cholesterol levels, and the FDA allows fiber products in foods to make claims for heart health.

Bulk laxatives have a slow onset of action and may take 1 to 3 days for maximum effect. Because they are replacing fiber normally consumed in the diet, they may be used for more than the 7 days period of use recommended for most other laxatives if the cause of constipation is lack of dietary fiber. Some of the causes of lack of dietary fiber are poor food choices by individuals, inability to chew foods that have a high fiber content, inability to digest fiber and/or the creation of intestinal gas, and the cost of some high fiber foods.

Warning and precautions

Taking bulk laxatives without adequate fluid may cause them to swell and block the throat or esophagus, causing choking. These products should not be taken by individuals who have difficulty swallowing. Immediate medical attention should be sought if chest pain, vomiting, or difficulty in swallowing or breathing is experienced after taking these products; if there is no bowel movement; or if abdominal discomfort and pain persist. Inadequate fluid intake while using bulk laxatives may lead to intestinal blockage or obstruction.[23]

The bulk laxatives should not be used when abdominal pain, nausea, or vomiting is present. If any blood appears in the stool or vomit, a physician must be consulted because self-care is not appropriate.

Cellulose and methylcellulose should not be taken without consulting a physician or pharmacist if an individual is taking salicylate drugs or prescription drugs because of possible drug interactions.

Recommended dosage

All powdered products should be mixed with at least 6 ounces (170 mL) of water or other fluid-like juices. If tablets or wafers containing bulk laxatives are used, they should be followed by an increased intake of fluids. Doses for bulk laxatives appear in table 3.5.

Table 3.5 Usual recommended doses for oral laxatives; all drugs are taken as one single dose in a day			
Drug	Over 12 years and adult	6–11 years	2–5 years
Bulk laxatives			
Bran	6–14 g	Consult doctor	Consult doctor
Methylcellulose	4–6 g	1–1.5 g	Consult doctor
Malt soup extract	12–64 g	12–64 g	12–64 g
Polycarbophil	4–6 g	1.5–3 g	1–1.5 g
Psyllium	2.5–30 g	1.25–15 g	Consult doctor
Lubricant laxatives			
Mineral oil	15–45 mL	5 mL	Consult doctor
Hyperosmotic/saline laxatives			
Magnesium citrate	11–25 g	5.5–12.5 g	2.7–6.25 g
Magnesium hydroxide (MOM)	2.4–4.8 g	1.2–2.4 g	0.4–1.2 g
Mixed sodium phosphates	20–45 mL	Age 10 & 11: 10–20 mL; age 5–9: 5–10 mL	Consult doctor
Stimulant (irritant) laxatives			
Bisacodyl	5–15 mg	5 mg	Consult doctor
Castor oil	15–60 mL	5–15 mL	5–15 mL
Senna (sennosides A and B)	12–50 mg	6–25 mg	3–12.5 mg
Stool softeners			
Docusate calcium	50–360 mg	50–150 mg	50–150 mg
Docusate sodium	50–360 mg	50–150 mg	50–150 mg
Osmotic laxative			
Polyethylene glycol (PEG) 3350	17 g restrict to age 18 and over	Consult doctor	Consult doctor

Products
Guar gum (Benefiber), malt soup extract (Maltsupex), methycellulose (Citrucel), polycarbophil (Equalactin), polycarbophil calcium (Fiber Con tablets, Konsyl Fiber caplets, and Perdiem fiber therapy caplets), and psyllium (Konsyl, Konsyl for Kids and Metamucil).

Lubricant laxatives

Drug category and indications for use
Plain mineral oil or emulsified mineral oil emulsions are monograph laxatives for short-term relief (1 week) of constipation.

Mode of action
Lubricant laxatives mix with the contents of the intestinal tract to make elimination of the stool easier.

Warnings and precautions
Lubricant laxatives should not be used in children under 6 years of age, in pregnant women, in bedridden or aged individuals, in individuals who have difficulty in swallowing, or individuals who are experiencing episodes of vomiting or abdominal pain. If an individual has a problem with fecal incontinence, leakage of stool through the anal sphincter may occur with use of mineral oil laxatives. Mineral oil products should not be used with stool softeners.[22]

Recommended dose
Emulsifier mineral may be administered during the day or at bedtime, but plain mineral oil should only be administered at bedtime. See table 3.5 for doses.

Products
Mineral oil (many generic manufacturers; Fleet Mineral Oil Enema), emulsified mineral oil (Kondremul). All enemas should be administered while the individual is lying on their left side.

Hyperosmotic and/or saline laxatives

Drug category and indications for use
Hyperosmotic and saline laxatives may be used occasionally for relief of constipation.

Mode of action
Hyperosmotic and saline laxatives greatly increase the osmotic pressure in the lumen of the intestinal tract and water is drawn into the intestine to equalize pressure. This causes a rapid response in stretch receptors that usually results in watery bowel movements.

Glycerin is classified as a hyperosmotic laxative and is restricted to rectal use. Magnesium citrate, magnesium hydroxide, magnesium and mixed phosphate salts (sodium phosphate and sodium biphosphate), all inorganic salts, are classified as saline laxatives and are administered orally. Mixed phosphate salts may also be used rectally.

Warnings and/precautions

Hyperosmotic and saline laxatives should not be used if abdominal pain, nausea, or vomiting is present. If any blood appears in the stool, a physician must be consulted because self-care is not appropriate.[22]

Excessive use of oral hyperosmotic laxatives may result in dehydration in individuals who do not maintain an adequate intake of daily fluids; this can lead to hospitalization and even death. The very young, the elderly, and generally frail individuals are at greatest risk for dehydration. An 8 ounce (230 mL) glass of fluid should be taken with every oral dose of a hyperosmotic drug.

Magnesium citrate solution should be stored in a cold place (refrigerator) to prevent degradation of the drug and to increase its palatability. Most hyperosmotic laxatives have a disagreeable taste, which may limit their usefulness. If the daily dose of magnesium exceeds 600 mg and the individual has kidney disease, a physician should be consulted before use.

If the individual has kidney disease, oral phosphate laxatives should not be used without the supervision of a physician. If the daily dose contains more than 115 mg of sodium, a physician should be consulted if the individual is on a low sodium diet. The FDA restricts the packaging of oral phosphate solution to 3 ounces (80 g) to prevent serious adverse effects.[24]

Oral phosphates were recommended frequently by physicians when a thorough bowel cleansing before colonoscopy or bowel surgery was required. The FDA issued a safety alert for both OTC and prescription oral phosphates use for bowel cleansing in December 2008. The FDA received reports of acute phosphate nephropathy and now requires a special warning on all oral phosphate prescription products.[25] The FDA alert does not affect the status of rectal phosphate products.

C.B. Fleet Laboratories, a major manufacturer of OTC oral phosphates solution (Phospho-Soda), voluntarily removed its oral products from the market except Fleet Phospho-Soda EZ Prep Bowel Cleansing. The FDA has not issued any recall for oral phosphate products, either OTC or prescription products. Some generic manufacturers may still have oral phosphate solutions on the market.

Glycerin is restricted to rectal use as a suppository or enema, and it may cause some rectal burning after insertion into the rectum.[22]

Recommended dose

Oral dosing for hyperosmotic drugs appears in table 3.5. Glycerin suppositories should not be used in children under 2 years of age unless supervised by a physician. Suppositories with 1 to 1.7 g glycerin may be used in children aged between 2 and 6 years and are inserted rectally. (These suppositories are referred to as infant suppositories.) Suppositories with 2 to 3 g of glycerin are intended for use in children over 6 years of age and for adults. Glycerin enemas containing 2 to 5 mL may be administered to children 2 to 5 years of age, and enemas with 5 to 15 mL of glycerin may be used in children age 6 years or over and in adults.

A daily dose of mixed phosphate enemas may contain approximately 7 g of dibasic sodium phosphate and 19 g of monobasic sodium biphosphate in 4 ounces (115 mL) of fluid for adults and children aged 12 years and older, and doses of 3.5 g and 9.5 g, respectively, in 2 ounces (58 mL) of fluid for children aged 2 to 11 years of age.[22]

Products
Glycerin suppositories and enemas (many generic manufacturers, Pedia-Lax Liquid Glycerin Suppositories (formerly named BabyLax), and Pedia-Lax Glycerin Suppositories), magnesium hydroxide (Philip's Milk of Magnesia, Freelax, and Pedia-Lax Chewable Tablets), and mixed phosphates (Fleet Saline Enema and Fleet Pedia-Lax Enema).

Stimulant laxatives (secretory or irritant) laxatives

Drug category and indications for use
Stimulant laxatives are for short-term relief (1 week) of occasional constipation.

Mode of action
Stimulant laxatives promote bowel movements by acting on the mucosal wall of the intestine, hence the name irritant. They may increase secretions into the intestine that stimulate stretch receptors to cause defecation, hence the name secretory or stimulant. Bisacodyl, castor oil, and senna are classified as stimulant laxatives. Castor oil acts on both the small and large intestine, causing a more watery bowel movement, and should not be recommended because it is more likely to cause dehydration than the other stimulant laxatives.

Warnings and precautions
Stimulant laxatives should not be used when abdominal pain, nausea, or vomiting is present. If any blood appears in the stool, a physician must be consulted because self-care is not appropriate.

Bisacodyl tablets are enteric coated and should not be crushed or chewed; they should not be taken with milk or within 1 hour of ingesting antacids or milk (dairy) products. Abdominal discomfort or cramps may occur, and burning may occur during defecation. The stimulant laxatives are stored at temperatures lower than 86°F (30°C).

Recommended dose

Oral doses for stimulant laxatives appear in table 3.5. Bisacodyl may be used as a single 10 mg suppository daily in children 6 to 12 years of age and in adults; a 5 mg suppository may be used daily in children between 2 and 5 years of age.

Products

Bisacodyl (Dulcolax tablets and suppositories, ExLax Ultra Stimulant Laxative, Correctol, and Carter's Laxative), senna (Senokot, ExLax Regular Chocolate, and Pedia-Lax Quick Dissolve Strips).

Stool softeners

Drug category and indications for use

Stool softeners are intended for short-term relief (1 week) of constipation unless supervised by a physician.

Many physicians recommend long-term use of stool softeners in geriatric patients or patients who requires opiates for pain. Docusate calcium, docusate potassium, and docusate sodium are classified as stool softeners.

Mode of action

Stool softeners act as surface active agents (detergents) that can penetrate dry, hard stools in the large intestine to soften the stool for easier elimination.

Warnings and precautions

Stool softeners should not be used when abdominal pain, nausea, or vomiting is present. If any blood appears in the stool, a physician must be consulted because self-care is not appropriate. Stool softeners should not be used with mineral oil or prescription drugs without consulting a healthcare professional.[22]

Special warnings for docusate potassium include: 'Do not use this drug if it contains more than 975 mg of potassium in the daily dose if you have kidney disease without supervision by a doctor.'

Special warnings for docusate sodium include: 'Do not use this drug if it contains more than 345 mg of sodium in the daily dose if you are on a low salt diet without supervision by a doctor; do not use this drug if you have kidney disease without supervision of a doctor.'

Recommended dose

See table 3.5.

Products

Docusate calcium (Kaopectate Stool Softener Liquigels), docusate potassium (generic products), and docusate sodium (Colace, Pedia-Lax Liquid Stool Softener, and Sof-Lax).

Carbon dioxide

Drug category and indications for use
Carbon dioxide suppositories are intended for short-term relief of constipation.

Mode of action
When suppositories containing sodium biphosphate (1.2 to 1.5 g), sodium acid phosphate (0.04 to 0.05 g), and sodium bicarbonate (1 to 1.5 g) or sodium bicarbonate (0.6 g) and potassium bitartrate (0.9 g) are used rectally, they produce a chemical reaction that releases carbon dioxide gas. The carbon dioxide gas expands, resulting in stimulation of stretch receptors to initiate a bowel movement.

Recommended dose
Adults and children age 12 years and over may insert one suppository rectally daily. The suppository should be moistened by dipping it in a cup of water for 10 seconds or holding it in under running water for at least 30 seconds before insertion into the rectum.[22]

Product
Carbon dioxide suppositories (Ceo-Two Suppositories).

Bowel preparation kits

Drug category and indications for use
Bowel preparation kits contain a combination of laxatives that are intended for use when medical procedures, such as colonoscopies and GI surgical procedures, are to be performed. These procedures require the large intestine be free of any fecal material. Physicians may use either prescription or OTC products, which are taken the day before the scheduled procedure for bowel cleansing. Only short-acting laxatives are used for the purpose.[22] These products are not to be used unless directed to do so by a physician.

Mode of action
OTC laxatives that have a fast onset of action may be used alone or in combinations. Saline laxatives (mixed phosphates and magnesium citrate) and stimulant laxatives (bisacodyl and sennosides) are used for this purpose. The mode of action for each appears earlier in this chapter. Oral phosphate products may still be used by physicians for bowel cleansing, but the new required labeling increase their awareness of the serious adverse effects to the kidneys from acute phosphate nephropathy.[25]

Recommended dose
The products are used according to a physician's directions as a bowel cleansing preparation.

Product
Mixed phosphates (Fleet Phospho-Soda EZ Prep Bowel Cleansing). This is the only Fleet oral phosphate product that remains on the OTC market at this time, but it may not be on shelves available for consumers' selection. Many pharmacists have this product available as a behind-the-counter product so that the consumers may be educated as to the proper use of the product and its potential for serious adverse effects before purchasing it.

Combination laxatives

The monograph permits two laxatives to be combined in a single product, providing that each laxative has a different mode of action.

Product
Senna and sodium docusate (PeriColace).

Osmotic laxatives

Drug category and indications for use
Polyethylene glycol 3350 (PEG 3350) is an osmotic laxative intended for temporary relief of constipation.[26]

Rx–OTC switched drug
Polyethylene glycol 3350.

Mode of action
An osmotic laxative draws water into the intestines to mix with its contents and cause swelling, thus initiating defecation. Unlike hyperosmotic laxatives, which have a very fast action, osmotic laxatives have a slow effect because of their lower osmolarity. While hyperosmotic laxatives are effective within hours, osmotic laxatives take 1 to 3 days to achieve their effect. This slower response also greatly reduces the possibility of dehydration and reduces the risk of causing abdominal gas and cramping.[26]

Warnings and precautions
If an individual has kidney disease, a physician should be contacted before using the drug. Osmotic laxatives should not be used for more than 7 days.

Recommended dose
PEG 3350 is taken once daily as 17 g (one cap full) added to 4 to 8 ounces (115–230 mL) of water or juice. It should not be used by individuals under 17 years of age.[26]

Product
PEG 3350 (MiraLax).

Antidiarrheal agents

When the contents of the intestines contain too much fluid, or movement through the GI tract is too rapid, fluids cannot be absorbed and an excessive volume reaches the large intestine. This results in sudden initiation of stretch receptors and rapid evacuation of the colon, causing diarrhea. Thus, diarrhea presents the opposite problems to those associated with constipation. When fluid balance and GI motility are restored, bowel movements return to a normal pattern. Diarrhea is usually defines as more than three loose or watery bowel movements per day without any known cause. This rapid movement of fluid through the GI tract is often accompanied by gas, cramping, or general abdominal discomfort.

Traveler's diarrhea is a common condition when an individual travels to areas with relatively poor sanitation. It is most commonly caused by ingestion of contaminated foods or water that contains fecal *Escherichia coli*, which produces an endotoxin, but other bacteria or viruses are also known to cause diarrhea. Uncooked foods and unpurified water should be avoided to lessen the risk of accidental ingestion of contaminated substances.

Diarrhea that is suspected of being caused by bacterial organisms, other than traveler's diarrhea, requires referral to a physician for proper diagnosis and treatment with prescription antibiotics. Diarrhea caused by viruses is frequently of short duration, and oral fluids should be used to prevent dehydration. Individuals who have profound diarrhea or diarrhea lasting more than 48 to 72 hours should consult a physician.

Ingestion of substances that can create increased osmotic pressure in the bowel may cause diarrhea if they are used in large quantities or for long periods of time. Magnesium-containing dietary supplements and xylitol, mannitol, and sorbitol sweeteners in candy, gums and foods are common substances that may cause diarrhea.

Adsorbants

Drug category and indications for use
Antidiarrheal drugs reduce or stop symptoms associated with diarrhea. Kaolin is the only monograph adsorbant and it helps to firm stools within 24 to 48 hours.[27]

Monograph ingredient
Kaolin suspension.

Mode of action
Adsorbant drugs adsorb water in the GI tract to create a semisolid mass, thus lessening the amount of fluid that reached the large intestine. This may both reduce the frequency of bowel movements and make them less watery.

Warnings and precautions

Adsorbant drugs should not be used without consulting a physician if stools are bloody or black or there is mucus in the stool, or if a fever is present. If other medications are being taken, kaolin should be taken either 3 hours before or 3 hours after the other drugs. A physician should be consulted if the diarrhea gets worse or if it lasts for more than 48 hours. Plenty of fluids should be drunk to prevent the dehydration caused by diarrhea.[27]

Electrolyte solutions or juices that do not contain an excess of glucose or sugar are better sources of fluid than plain water. Caffeine and alcoholic drinks should be avoided because they cause excess urination with additional fluid loss.

Recommended dose

Adults and children over 12 years of age should take 26 g of the product after each loose bowel movement or every 6 hours; it should not be taken for more than 2 days. Children under 12 years of age should not take the product without the supervision of a physician.[27]

Products

Kaolin suspension (generic products).

Bismuth subsalicylate

Drug category and indications for use

Bismuth subsalicylate may be used to control or relieve the symptoms of diarrhea or traveler's diarrhea; it reduces the number of bowel movements and helps to firm stools.[28]

Mode of action

Bismuth subsalicylate is an astringent and coats the mucosa. It produces some effect because it has adsorbant properties, but it also has antisecretory effects, which reduces the amount of fluids entering the GI tract.

Warning and precautions

Bismuth subsalicylate should not be used without consulting a physician if stools are bloody or black, if there is mucus in the stool, or if a fever is present. There may be a temporary darkening of the tongue and stools from use of this drug.

Bismuth subsalicylate does not contain aspirin, but it may cause an adverse effect in an individual allergic to aspirin; it should not be used in children or teenagers who have or are recovering from chickenpox or flu-like symptoms (Reye's syndrome warning); those taking anticoagulants (blood thinning drugs) should consult their physician before use.

Those with diabetes, gout, or arthritis should ask a physician or pharmacist before using this product. If ringing in the ears or a loss of hearing develops, stop using the drug. If symptoms get worse or diarrhea last for more than 48 hours, a physician should be consulted. Plenty of fluids should be drunk to prevent dehydration caused by diarrhea.[28]

Recommended dose
Adults and children over 12 years of age may take 1050 mg bismuth subsalicylate every 30 to 60 minutes but should not exceed 4200 mg in 24 hours; bismuth subsalicylate should not be used for more than 2 days. Children aged 9 to 11 years may take one-half the adult dose (525 mg); children aged 6 to 8 years may take 350 mg; children aged 3 to 6 years may take one-sixth of the adult dose (175 mg); children under 3 years of age require recommendation by physician.[28]

Products
Bismuth subsalicylate (Pepto-Bismol, Kaopectate).

Loperamide

Drug category and indications
Loperamide is an anticholinergic drug that is used to reduce or stop diarrhea, including traveler's diarrhea.[29]

Rx–OTC switched drug
Loperamide.

Mode of action
Anticholinergic drugs block the action of the peripheral parasympathetic nervous system and reduce GI motility. This allows more time for absorption of fluid from the GI tract and reduces the watery stools.

Warnings and precautions
Loperamide should not be used for more than 48 hours or in individuals who have an elevated body temperature greater than 101°F (38.3°C); use of this drug may cause a rash. Loperamide should not be used in children under 6 years of age.[29]

Recommended dose
The dose of loperamide for adults and children aged 12 years and over is 4 mg after the first loose bowel movement and 2 mg after each loose bowel movement thereafter. The maximum daily dose is 8 mg.

Children between 6 and 11 years of age may take 2 mg after the first loose bowel movement and 1 mg after each loose bowel movement thereafter. The maximum daily dose is 4 mg. When the liquid formulation is used, the measuring device in the packaging should be used for exact measure for children's doses.

Products
Loperamide (Imodium A–D), loperamide with simethicone (Imodium Multi-symptom Relief). The combination of simethicone and loperamide is permitted because gas and abdominal distention occur frequently in individuals who have diarrhea.

Lactose intolerance

Individuals who lack the enzyme lactase are not able to digest lactose, a sugar common in milk and milk products. This causes symptoms of gas, bloating, and diarrhea. Because lactose is not metabolized, it increases the osmotic pressure in the intestines and, therefore, acts as a hyperosmotic laxative.

Eliminating lactose from the diet, or consuming it in small quantities will generally prevent symptoms. Because a relatively large portion of the US population has lactose intolerance, foods that have reduced lactose or are lactose free are available in food markets. These include Lactaid Free Milk, Dairy Ease Fat Free Milk, and soy milk products. Another alternative to solving this problem relies on providing lactase enzyme as a dietary supplement or a food by using products such as Lactaid. The FDA is considering classifying lactase as an OTC drug but has not done so at this time.

Probiotics

The human GI tract contains a variety of bacteria known collectively as 'gut flora'; these have several important functions in the body, such as synthesizing vitamin K and helping to maintain normal bowel balance and function. Bouts of noninfectious diarrhea deplete the GI tract of these bacteria. The use of oral preparations containing live strains of normal gut flora, probiotics, assists in repopulating the GI tract, reducing the duration of diarrhea, and possibly preventing other episodes of diarrhea. Individuals who are prescribed antibiotic drugs that affect a wide range of bacteria, including gut flora, often develop diarrhea.

Lactobacillus and *Bifidobacterium* are the two most common species of nonpathogenic bacteria used as probiotics; *Saccharomyces boulardii*, a yeast, is another popular probiotic. The efficacy of the various strains of *Lactobacillus* vary, and those with the most positive results in published studies are *L. acidophilus*, *L. bulgarius*, *L. casei*, and *L. reuteri*. Several of these species are present in yogurts, fermented milk and soy milk.[30] Preparations of these bacteria are available in capsule form and as granules. The FDA regulates these products as dietary supplements and foods, not OTC drugs.

Products
Lactobacillus (Cultrelle, Probiotica), Bifidobacterium (Align), Saccharomyces (Florastor).

Electrolyte solutions

The excessive watery stools that occur during diarrhea may result in dehydration. Several OTC electrolyte solutions are available to help to prevent the loss of both fluid volume and electrolytes during diarrhea. Most products are formulated based on the recommendations of the World Health Organization (WHO) oral rehydration solutions. Apple juice, other fruit juices, and carbonated beverages may contain a high quantity of carbohydrates and should be avoided. Such high-carbohydrate drinks could worsen diarrhea because of they would increase osmotic pressure in the GI tract, thus acting as osmotic laxatives.

Products
Oral electrolyte products (Pedialyte and CeraLyte). Gatorade, a food product, contains electrolytes and is a good substitute as a source of fluids instead of fruit juices.

Miscellaneous products

Internal oral deodorants

Drug category and indications for use
Individuals who have ostomies (ileostomy or colostomy) or urinary and fecal incontinence experience difficulty with control of odors.[31]

Monograph ingredients
Chlorophyllin copper complex, bismuth subgallate.

Mode of action
No specific test for efficacy or mode of action is given in the FDA monograph that recognizes chlorophyllin copper complex and bismuth subgallate as monograph ingredients to help to reduce odor problems resulting from ostomies or incontinence problems. Individuals who have odor problems should also avoid foods that are likely to cause odors, such as fish, eggs, garlic, onions, and asparagus. Vitamin products and some prescription antibiotics also cause odor problems.

Warnings and precautions
If cramps or diarrhea occur with chlorophyllin copper complex, the recommended dose should be reduced; if symptoms continue, consult your physician.

Recommended dose
Chlorophyllin copper complex may be used by adults and children 12 years of age or older in doses of 100 mg but should not exceed 300 mg per day.

Bismuth subgallate may be used by adults and children 12 years of age or older in doses of 200 to 400 mg up to four times a day.

Products

Chlorophyllin copper complex (Nullo), bismuth subgallate (Devrom).

Case study exercises

Case 1 GM, *a 57-year-old male, was treated for gastric ulcers last year and hasn't had a prescription for a proton pump inhibiting drug for the last 4 months. He asks the pharmacist whether he should take PrilosecOTC or Zantac 150 mg because he has been experiencing heartburn symptoms once a week for the past 3 weeks.*

GM's heartburn problem does not fit the criteria for use of PrilosecOTC, which is frequent heartburn, two or more times a week. However, because of his history of gastric ulcers he may be experiencing a recurrence of ulcer disease. The pharmacist advises him to make an appointment with his doctor and to use Zantac to relieve his symptoms until he sees his doctor.

Case 2 *The mother of a 10-year-old child who just recovered from chickenpox asks the pharmacist if Pepto Bismol is a good product to relieve the child's upset stomach. The mother says that the child has no health problems and is not taking any type of medication except a daily vitamin, which has never seemed to cause any problem.*

The pharmacist advises the mother to avoid Pepto Bismol because it contains a salicylate. Aspirin and salicylate products should not be used in children who have had chickenpox or flu because of their association with Reye's syndrome. The pharmacist recommends a calcium carbonate antacid such as Mylanta Children's chewable tablets. The mother should be advised to contact the doctor if the child's symptoms are not relieved within a day or two.

Case 3 JL, *a 26-year-old female, asks the pharmacist if Regular Alka-Seltzer is suitable for use for an upset stomach and hangover she has from a weekend of partying that included a lot of food and alcoholic beverages.*

The pharmacist advises JL that sodium bicarbonate, which is in regular Alka-Seltzer, is contraindicated for use when overindulgence is the problem. Alka-Seltzer Wake-up Call, any of the other antacids and Pepto Bismol are suitable for her symptoms.

Case 4 SB *is a 60-year-old man who has a history of motion sickness. He tells the pharmacist that the Dramamine that he has been using now*

makes him very drowsy. He wants to know if there is a better product for him to use. His only other medical problem is hypertension.
The pharmacist recommends that he try motion sickness products that contain either cyclizine or meclizine, because they usually cause less drowsiness than dimenhydrinate, the active ingredient in Dramamine. He should be cautioned that these products also have to potential to cause drowsiness.

Case 5 A pregnant woman who has 'morning sickness' symptoms asks the pharmacist to recommend a product for her symptoms.
The pharmacist tells her that OTC drugs are not approved by the FDA for use in pregnant women without supervision by a doctor. She should also ask her doctor about the possible use of ginger, a food additive and a dietary supplement, because there is evidence that it is of some benefit in relieving nausea associated with pregnancy (See also p. 45).

Case 6 CY is a 45-year-old business man who has returned from a 6 day trip to China. He explains that he normally has a daily bowel movement but that he hasn't had one in 4 days and his abdomen feels full and uncomfortable.
The pharmacist recommends using a stimulant laxative like bisacodyl or senna to relieve his constipation. If he doesn't get relief from these symptoms, he should consult his doctor. A single dose of a hyperosmotic such as magnesium citrate or milk of magnesia is a suitable alternative. A laxative suppository or enema could also be recommended, but these formulations are less likely to be used than oral laxatives.

Case 7 LM got new dentures (false teeth) 3 weeks ago and has been eating soft foods and soups because she still has discomfort in chewing foods. Her regular bowel movements have decreased from every other day to about twice a week.
The pharmacist recommends that she increase bulk in her diet by using a bulk laxative such as psyllium, bran, or methylcellulose. She should also drink more fluids, especially if she chooses to use one of these products. If she doesn't have relief from her symptoms, she should consult her doctor.

Case 8 A 45-year-old woman asks the pharmacist for Fleet's Phospho-Soda EZ Prep Bowel Cleansing because her doctor recommended it.
The pharmacist discusses this purchase with the individual and learns that she is having a colonoscopy in 2 days and this product is part of her

preparation for the procedure. The pharmacist explains that the Phospho-Soda product must be taken exactly as directed by her physician and must be taken with the recommended amount of fluid because dehydration and possible kidney damage may occur if directions are not followed.

Case 9 KG has three children between 3 and 9 years old and one of them has pinworms. She asks the pharmacist what to do.
The pharmacist tells her that everyone in the family, including all the adults, should take a single dose of pryantel pamoate, and the dose is based on body weight, 11 mg per kilogram (5 mg per pound). The pharmacist also outlines cleaning and sanitary measures that must be followed to prevent reoccurrence.

Case 10 A mother complains that her 5-year-old child has had diarrhea for 3 days and won't eat or drink. She asks the pharmacist if loperamide (Imodium AD) by itself or combined with simethicone (Imodium Multi-symptom) is better.
The pharmacist tells her to call the doctor immediately because diarrhea lasting for more than 48 hours without appropriate fluid intake could lead to dehydration that must be managed by a doctor. She should continue try to get the child to drink fluids. Loperamide is not approved for use in children under 6 years of age and, therefore, neither product should be used.

Case 11 KT has just returned from South America and is experiencing diarrhea from fresh, unwashed fruit he bought at the airport. What should he do?
The pharmacist recommends drinking fluids and using either loperamide or bismuth subsalicylate according to the labeled directions. If relief does not occur within 48 hours, he should consult his doctor.

References

1. Antacid products and antiflatulents for over-the-counter (OTC) human use; final monograph. *Fed Regist* 1974; 39: 19862–19877.
2. Orally administered drug products for relief of symptoms associated with overindulgence in food and drink for over-the-counter human use; tentative final monograph; notice of proposed rulemaking. *Fed Regist* 1991; 56: 66742–66751. www.fda.gov/cder/otcmonographs/category_sort/overindulgence (accessed November 12, 2008).
3. Antacid drug products for over-the-counter human use; Proposed Amendment of Antacid Final Monograph. *Fed Regist* 1994; 59: 5060–5065.

4. Antacid drug products for over-the-counter human use; amendment of antacid final monograph; technical amendment. *Fed Regist* 1994; 59: 60555–60556.

5. Orally administered drug products for relief of symptoms associated with overindulgence in food and drink for over-the-counter human use; proposed amendment of the tentative final monograph. *Fed Regist* 2005; 70: 741–746. www.fda.gov/cder/otcmonographs/category_sort/overindulgence (accessed November 12, 2008).

6. Pepto Bismol. www.pepto-bismol.com/index.php (accessed November 18, 2008).

7. Tagamet. www.tagamethb.com/faqs.aspx (accessed November 17, 2008).

8. *Questions and answers on Prilosec OTC (Omeprazole)*. www.fda.gov/cder/drug/infopage/prilosecOTC/prilosecotcQ&A.htm (accessed November 17, 2008).

9. Cohen-Silver J, Ratnapalan S. Management of infantile colic. *Clin Pediatr (Phil)* 2009; 48: 14–17.

10. Mylicon. www.mylicon.com (accessed November 28, 2008).

11. Beanogas. www.Beanogas.com/UsingBeano.aspx (accessed November 17, 2008).

12. Kligler B, Chaudhary S. Peppermint oil. *Am Fam Physician* 2007; 75: 1027–1030.

13. Antiemetic drug products for over-the-counter human use: final rule. *Fed Regist* 1987; 52: 15886–15891.

14. White B. Ginger: an overview. *Am Fam Physician* 2007; 75: 1689–1691.

15. Emetrol. www.brands2liveby.com/product.aspx?id=407 (accessed November 18, 2008).

16. Acupressure. http://altmed.creighton.edu/Ginger/Acupressure.htm (accessed May 26, 2009).

17. Relief Band. www.ReliefBand.com/answers.html (accessed May 26, 2009).

18. Manoguerra AS, Cobaugh DJ. Guideline on the use of ipecac syrup in the out-of-hospital management of ingested poisons. *Clin Toxic* (Phila) 2005; 43: 1–10.

19. Miscellaneous internal drug products for over-the-counter human use. Sub Part A: Poison treatment drug products. *Fed Regist* 1985; 50: 2259–2262.

20. Anthelmintic drug products for over-the-counter human use; final monograph. *Fed Regist* 1986; 51: 27756–27760.

21. Costanzo LS. *Physiology*, 3rd edn. Philadelphia, PA: Elsevier, 2006: 327–375.

22. Laxative drug products for over-the-counter human use; tentative final monograph. *Fed Regist* 1985; 50: 2124–2158. www.fda.gov/cder/otcmonographs/Laxative/new_laxative.htm (accessed November 14, 2008).

23. Warning statements required for over-the-counter drugs containing water-soluble gums as active ingredients. *Fed Regist* 1993; 58: 45194–45201. www.fda.gov/cder/otcmonographs/Laxative/new_laxative.htm (accessed November 14, 2008).

24. Package size limitation for sodium phosphates oral solution and warning and direction statements for oral and rectal sodium phosphates for over-the-counter laxative use. *Fed Regist* 1998; 63: 27836–27843. www.fda.gov/cder/otcmonographs/Laxative/new_laxative.htm (accessed November 14, 2008).

25. Oral sodium phosphate (OSP) products for bowel cleansing (marketed as Visicol and OsmoPrep, and oral sodium phosphate products available without prescription). www.fda.gov/cder/drug/infopage/OSP_solution/default.htm (accessed May 20, 2009).

26. drugstore. www.drugstore.com/products/prod.asp?pid=172404&catid=172 (accessed November 17, 2008).

27. Antidiarrheal drug products for over-the-counter human use: final monograph. *Fed Regist* 2003; 68: 18869–18882. www.fda.gov/cder/otcmonographs/Antidiarrheal/new_antidiarrheal.htm (accessed December 1, 2008).

28. Over-the-counter drug products; safety and efficacy review; additional antidiarrheal ingredient. *Fed Regist* 2004; 69: 51852–51853.

29. Imodium. www.imodium.com/page.jhtml/?id=imodium/include/2_0.inc (accessed December 2, 2008).

30. Floch MH *et al.* Recommendations for probiotic use: 2008. *J Clin Gastrol* 2008; 42(Suppl 2): S104–S108 .

31. Deodorant drug products for internal use for over-the-counter human use; final monograph. *Fed Regist* 1990; 55: 19862–19866.

4

Respiratory system

This chapter outlines the management of common respiratory symptoms that affect either the upper respiratory or lower respiratory system. The upper respiratory system includes the nose, throat, and sinuses. Allergies, the common cold, flu (influenza), and rhinosinusitis have many of the same symptoms and many drugs may be used in the treatment of these conditions. Antihistamines and decongestants are the most commonly used drugs for all these conditions. Some individuals may have headache or sinus discomfort and pain, and OTC analgesics (see Chapter 5) may also be useful. These drugs may used alone or combined in a single product.

The common cold and flu have additional symptoms, including coughs, chest congestion, fever, and possible myalgia (muscle aches). Antitussives (cough suppressants), expectorants, and antipyretics address these symptoms, and they may be used alone or in combinations. All of the treatments for the common cold and flu are symptomatic and provided limited relief. Several dietary supplements and homeopathic products are very popular for treating colds or flu, but there are few controlled clinical trials providing evidence of their efficacy.

The lower respiratory system includes the trachea, bronchial tubes, and lungs. The FDA only approved products for use in patients who have asthma, provided that they had been previously diagnosed as having asthma by a physician.

Allergies

Rhinorrhea (runny nose), nasal congestion, and sinusitis are symptoms associated with allergic conditions and upper respiratory infections. Proper treatment requires differentiation based on onset, duration, and severity of symptoms plus the presence of additional symptoms such as fever or headache.

Antihistamines

Drug category and indications for use

Antihistamines (H_1-blockers or histamine antagonists) relieve the symptoms of seasonal allergies (hay fever) and other upper respiratory allergies. They temporarily reduce runny nose and relieve sneezing, itching of the nose or throat, and itchy, watery eyes.[1]

Mode of action

Allergens (pollen, animal dandruff, foods, chemicals) produce changes that are most noticeable in the upper respiratory track or the skin. Allergens bind with immunoglobulin E (IgE) present in tissues and this reacts with surface receptors on mast cells and basophils to cause the release of histamine, tryptase, cysteinyl-leukotrienes, prostaglandin D, and cytokines (interleukins). These inflammatory mediators cause changes in capillary permeability, resulting in vasodilatation of blood vessels, edema, and thin, watery secretions of the nose and eyes, and/or a rash or hives.[2]

The best and safest method to prevent symptoms from allergic reactions is to avoid the allergen. Pharmacological treatment involves the use of oral antihistamines. All antihistamines have the same mode of action. They occupy the same receptors as histamine but do not cause its consequences, thereby preventing or minimizing symptoms. Their onset of action may be delayed if taken after symptoms occur because both histamine and the antihistamine compete for the same receptor sites.

The hallmark symptoms of rhinitis are copious, thin, watery nasal secretions, accompanied by itching, sneezing, and tearing, itchy eyes. Because the lining of the paranasal sinuses are usually affected, the term rhinosinusitis is frequently used instead of rhinitis. Rhinosinusitis may be allergic or non-allergic (vasomotor rhinitis of unknown origin, rhinitis associated with pregnancy, and rhinitis associated with aging are not associated with IgE release) and may be acute or chronic.[3]

Monograph drugs (first-generation, nonselective, or sedating antihistamines)

Mode of action

The first-generation monograph drugs cause drowsiness to a varying degree depending on their specific chemical structure. They possess some lipid solubility and are able to cross the blood–brain barrier to produce their sedative effect.[1] The alkylamine antihistamines include brompheniramine maleate and its dextro form, chlorpheniramine maleate and its dextro form, and triprolidine hydrochloride; these produce less sedation than the ethanolamine-type drugs. The ethanolamine antihistamines include diphenhydramine hydrochloride and citrate, doxylamine succinate, and clemastine fumarate.

All of these antihistamines have anticholinergic activity, contributing to the reduction of secretions and providing a rationale for their use in cough/cold products.

Warnings and precautions
These products should not be taken for more than 7 days unless directed by a physician. They should not be taken except under the advice and supervision of a physician by those with asthma, narrow-angle glaucoma, or difficulty urinating owing to enlargement of the prostate gland. These antihistamines may cause drowsiness (alcohol, sedatives, and tranquilizers may increase drowsiness) and should be used with caution when driving a motor vehicle or operating machinery. They may cause excitability, especially in children.[1]

Recommended doses
Dosages for antihistamines are given in table 4.1.

Products
Chlorpheniramine (ChlorTrimeton Allergy), clemastine (Tavist Allergy), diphenhydramine (Benadryl Allergy).

Rx–OTC switched drugs (second generation, peripherally selective or nonsedating antihistamines)

Cetirizine and loratadine are the only antihistamines currently available as OTC drugs in this category. Fexofenadine (Allegra) is a candidate for a future Rx–OTC switch.

Table 4.1 Recommended doses for antihistamines

Drug	Adult dose (dosing frequency)	6–12 years (dosing frequency)	2–5 years (dosing frequency)
Brompheniramine	4 mg (4–6 h)	2 mg (4–6 h)	1 mg (4–6 h)
Cetirizine	10 mg (24 h); > 65 years, 5 mg (24 h)	5–10 mg (24 h)	2.5 mg (24 h)
Chlorpheniramine	4 mg (4–6 h)	2 mg (4–6 h)	1 mg (4–6 h)
Clemastine	1 mg (12 h)	Consult physician	Consult physician
Diphenhydramine	25–50 mg (4–6 h)	12.5–25 mg (4–6 h)	Consult physician
Loratadine	10 mg daily	10 mg daily	5 mg daily
Triprolidine	2.5 mg (4–6 h)	1.25 mg (4–6 h)	4–5 years, 0.938 mg (4–6 h); 2–3 years, 0.625 mg (4–6 h)

Mode of action
Cetirizine and loratadine bind to the receptor site for histamine in the same manner as the FDA monograph antihistamines. They have less lipid solubility, greatly reducing or preventing penetration into the brain and producing less sedation. Both drugs lack the anticholinergic activity of the monograph antihistamines. They are available as tablets that dissolve on the tongue, providing an advantage over regular tablet formulations.

Warnings and precautions
Cetirizine should not be used if an individual is allergic to hydroxyzine. Cetirizine hydrochloride may cause drowsiness but it is much less severe than with the first-generation antihistamines. Cetirizine products intended for adults include a warning that individuals over the age of 65 years should consult a physician before using this drug.[4] However, labeling for cetirizine children's tablets and syrups, which contains 5 mg of cetirizine per dose, recommends that adults over 65 years may take one dose per day.[4] This is somewhat confusing because adults would not ordinarily choose a product intended for children for their use. The only adult products marketed at this time are 10 mg tablets that cannot be broken in half. The dose of cetrizine for adults over 65 is 5 mg once daily and, therefore, is only available in children's formulations at this time.

Cetirizine and loratadine should not be used without supervision of a physician if the individual has kidney or liver disease.[4,5]

Products
Cetirizine (Zyrtec, Children's Zyrtec Chewable Tablets, Children's Zyrtec Allergy Syrup, and Children's Zyrtec Hives Relief Syrup), loratadine (Alavert, Claritin, Claritin Hives Relief, Dimetapp Non-Drowsy Allergy, Tavist ND, and Triaminic Allerchews).

Mast cell inhibitors

Mode of action
Nasal cromolyn sodium prevents the release of histamine from mast cells in the presence of allergens. It must be used every 4 to 6 hours and is most effective if used before exposure; it should be used continuously during exposure.[6] Maximum relief occurs after 1 to 2 weeks of use. Cromolyn sodium is safe to use by individuals who should avoid antihistamines and it is a safe for use in children.

Warnings and precautions
Local irritation of nasal membranes may occur. Cromolyn sodium should not be used for treating asthma, colds, rhinosinusitis, or if a fever or nasal discharge is present.

Recommended dose

One spray is used in each nostril every 4 to 6 hours, but not more than 6 times a day. Cromolyn sodium should not be used in children under 2 years of age.

Products

Cromolyn sodium (NasalCrom and BenaMist).

Decongestants

Oral decongestants

Drug category and indications for use

Decongestants are vasoconstrictors that relieve nasal congestion from all causes of allergic or non-allergic rhinitis, the common cold, and other upper respiratory conditions including sinusitis.[7]

Monograph ingredients

Only phenylephrine and pseudoephedrine are available as OTC oral decongestants.[7] Because pseudoephedrine can be used to make methamphetamine, it is only available from the pharmacist. Some states permit sales of pseudoephedrine by a pharmacist or persons specifically trained by pharmacists. Individuals must have photo identification, be 18 years of age or older, and sign a register in order to purchase any product containing pseudoephedrine.[8]

Phenylepherine replaced pseudoephedrine in most OTC oral decongestant products. There is concern that the recommended minimum dose of 10 mg for adults may lack effectiveness and the FDA is reviewing this dosing issue.

Mode of action

The nasal passages have a very extensive blood supply, and neuropeptides released during the allergic or inflammatory process produce profound vasodilatation, causing nasal congestion. Oral or topical vasoconstrictors effectively relieve this nasal congestion.[2]

Warnings and precautions

Decongestants may cause nervousness, dizziness, or insomnia and should not be taken for more than 7 days. If symptoms do not improve or if a fever is present, a physician should be consulted. Decongestants should not be taken without consulting a physician by those with heart disease, high blood pressure, thyroid disease, diabetes, or with difficulty in urinating owing to prostate enlargement. They should not be taken with monoamine oxidase inhibiting drugs (MAOIs) used for hypertension or depression (phenelizine, tranylcypromine, isocarboxazid) or certain anti-Parkinson medications (e.g. selegiline and rasagiline).[7]

Table 4.2 Recommended doses for decongestants for allergies

Drug	Adult dose (dosing frequency)	6–12 years (dosing frequency)	2–5 years (dosing frequency)[a]
Oral			
Phenylephrine	10 mg (4 h)	5 mg (4 h)	2.5 mg (4 h)
Pseudoephedrine	60 mg (4–6 h)	30 mg (4–6 h)	15 mg (4–6 h)
Topical			
Levmetamfetamine	2 inhalations (2 h)	1 inhalation (2 h)	Consult physician
Oxymetazoline spray or drops	0.05% (10–12 h)	0.05% (10–12 h)	0.025% (10–12 h)
Phenylephrine spray or drops	0.25%, 0.5%, 1% (4 h)	0.25% (4 h)	0.125% (4 h)
Propylhexedrine	2 inhalations (2 h)	2 inhalations (2 h)	Consult physician

[a] No recommended doses for children under 4 years of age if decongestants are included in cough/cold products.

Recommended dose
Dosages for decongestants appear in table 4.2.

Products
Pseudoephedrine (Sudafed), phenylephrine (Sudafed PE).

Topical nasal decongestants

Drug category and indications for use
Topical nasal decongestants are available as nasal drops, sprays, or inhalers, and produce a quicker response than oral products. Overuse may cause rebound congestion, commonly referred to as rhinitis medicamentosa.[7]

Monograph ingredients
Topical nasal decongestants include levmetamfetamine, naphazoline hydrochloride, oxymetazoline, phenylepherine hydrochloride, and propylhexadrine, xylometazoline.

Mode of action
Topical nasal decongestants have the same vasoconstricting action on blood vessels as oral decongestants but they have an immediate onset of action.

Warnings and precautions
In addition to the warnings for oral decongestants, topical products may cause nasal irritation, stinging, sneezing, or increased nasal discharge. The FDA's labeling restricts the use to 3 days to prevent rebound congestion. Products for children should only be used with adult supervision.

Levmetamfetamine and propylhexadrine become vapors at normal temperature and should be tightly closed after use; they should only be used for 3 months once they are opened.

Recommended dose
Table 4.2 has dosage recommendations.

Products
Levmetamfetamine (Vicks Vapor Inhaler), oxymetazoline hydrochloride (Afrin, Vicks Sinex 12 Hour Nasal Spray, Zicam Intense Sinus Relief Nasal Spray), phenylephrine hydrochloride (Neo-Synephrine, Vicks Sinex for Sinus Relief), and propylhexadrine (Benzedrex Nasal Inhaler).

Nasal saline irrigation and cleansing

Mode of action
The discomfort accompanying nasal congestion may be relieved by the use of saline nasal sprays or drops, saline irrigation, or antimicrobial sprays. These products cleanse, moisturize, and soothe irritated nasal membranes. They are safe for use by patients who have conditions that preclude the use of decongestants, including women who are pregnant or breast feeding.

Warnings and precautions
Nasal sprays and drops should not be used in children without adult supervision.

Recommended dose
One or two sprays or drops are used in each nostril when needed.

Products
Ayr, Afrin Non-medicated, Little Noses, NaSal, Ocean, Pretz, Saline X, and Simply Soothing For Child & Baby Nose.

Neti pots are a popular nasal irrigation system. They contain a reservoir for either water or saline solution. The individual leans over a sink, tilts the head, and pours the solution into one nostril and allows it to drain out of the other nostril. Irritation of the nasal passages may result from this procedure.

Antimicrobial sprays

Mode of action
Cetylpyridinium is an effective antiseptic against bacteria, but its primary effect in treating nasal congestion and discomfort is by soothing dry and irritated membranes.

Warnings and precautions
Cetylpyridinium should not be used if nose bleeding is present. It should not be used for more than 7 days and if the symptoms do not improve, or get worse during use, a physician should be consulted.

Recommended dose
One to three sprays is used in each nostril twice a day. Cetylpyridinium should not be used for children under 12 years of age.

Product
Cetylpyridinium (SinoFresh)

External nasal dilator strips

Mode of action
An adhesive strip is applied to dry skin on each side of the nose. This device keeps the nostrils open, improving breathing in patients who have nasal congestion.[9] These devices may be safely used by individuals who cannot use decongestants, including women who are pregnant or breast feeding. Use of these nasal strips may be helpful in reducing snoring.

Warnings and precautions
These strips should not be used on irritated or broken skin and should be removed after 12 hours. Irritation from the adhesive may occur. The strips contain latex and should not be used by individuals who have latex allergies.

Products
Breathe Right, Breath Right for kids (ages 5 to 12), Breath Right with Menthol, Breatheasy, and Clear Passage.

Combination allergy drug therapy

Patients who have rhinitis, rhinosinusitis, or the common cold frequently experience rhinorrhea, sneezing, nasal congestion, and headache or sinus pain at the same time. Hence, the FDA permits numerous different drug combination products.[10]

Antihistamine and decongestant products
Alavert Allergy and Sinus, Allerest PE, Claritin D, Drixoral Cold and Allergy, Sudafed Sinus and Allergy, Triaminic Cold and Allergy, and Dimetapp Cold and Allergy.

Antihistamines and analgesic (usually acetaminophen) products
Coricidin HBP Cold and Flu, and Tylenol Severe Allergy. (These products are suitable for patients who must avoid decongestants, especially patients with hypertension, hyperthyroid and/or diabetes mellitus, a very large segment of the US population.)

Decongestants and analgesics products
Advil Cold and Sinus Non-drowsy, Alka Seltzer Plus Cold and Sinus, DayQuil Sinus, Sudafed Non-drowsy Sinus, and Tylenol Sinus Congestion and Pain Daytime. (Products containing the word 'non-drowsy', generally do not contain any antihistamine.)

Antihistamine, decongestant, and analgesic products
Advil Allergy and Sinus, Benadryl Allergy and Cold, Dristan Cold, NyQuil Sinus, and Tylenol Sinus Congestion and Pain Night Time.

Common cold

The common cold is an upper respiratory tract infection, usually caused by rhinoviruses or coronaviruses in adults. Parainfluenza virus and respiratory syncytial virus are additional causes in children. Most colds are self-limiting, lasting approximately 7 to 10 days, and treatment is purely symptomatic.

Viruses bind to intracellular adhesion molecule (ICAM-1) in the nasopharynx, initiating the release of the same inflammatory neuropeptides produced by allergens and causing the same upper respiratory symptoms.[2] Irritation of the throat from a postnasal drip associated with blockage of the nasal sinuses, which frequently accompanies colds, results in a nonproductive cough. Cough is the major symptom that distinguishes colds from other causes of rhinosinusitis.[11] A sore throat (pharyngitis) and occasionally a mild fever or headache may occur. Colds are differentiated from influenza (viral flu) infections by the severe fatigue and generalized muscle aches and pain that accompany flu infections.

Antitussives

Antitussives may provide mild, temporary symptomatic relieve by reducing or suppressing nonproductive coughs.[12]

Coughing is a protective mechanism to eliminate irritating substances or mucus from the lower respiratory tract. Cilia that line the airways move the irritants upward until they reach the pharynx, where they are eliminated by swallowing or expectorating (spitting). Individuals with lower respiratory tract infections must cough to maintain clear airways and lungs and remove excessive mucus to reduce the risk of pneumonia. This is a productive cough and should not be suppressed nor self-treated.

Central acting antitussives

Mode of action
Oral antitussive drugs produce their effect by suppressing the cough center in the brain.[12] Codeine compounds, dextromethorphan, and diphenhydramine are central-acting antitussives.[12] Because of the potential for abuse of codeine,

Table 4.3 Recommended doses for antitussives, expectorants and bronchodilators

Drug	Adult dose (dosing frequency)	6–12 years (dosing frequency)	2–5 years (dosing frequency)
Oral antitussives			
Codeine	10–20 mg (4–6 h)	12.5 mg (4–6 h)	Consult physician
Dextromethorphan	30 mg (6–8 h)	15 mg (6–8 h)	7.5 mg (6–8 h)[a]
Diphenhydramine HCl	25 mg (4 h)	12.5 mg (4 h)	Consult physician
Topical antitussives			
Camphor ointment	4.7–5.3% (3 times a day)	4.7–5.3% (3 times a day)	4.7–5.3% (3 times a day)
Menthol ointment	2.6–2.8% (3 times a day)	2.6–2.8% (3 times a day)	2.6–2.8% (3 times a day)
Menthol lozenge	5–10 mg (every hour)	5–10 mg (every hour)	5–10 mg (every hour)
Camphor steam	6.2% (3 times a day)	6.2% (3 times a day)	6.2% (3 times a day)
Menthol steam	3.2% (3 times a day)	3.2% (3 times a day)	3.2% (3 times a day)
Expectorants			
Guaifenesin	200–400 mg (4 h)	100–200 (4 h)	50–100 mg (4 h)[a]
Bronchodilators			
Ephedrine	12.5–25 mg (4 h)	Consult physician	Consult physician
Epinephrine 1% spray	1–3 inhalations (3 h)	1–3 inhalations (3 h)	4–6 years, 1–3 inhalations (3 h)

[a] No recommended doses for children under 4 years of age for use in cough/cold products.

a narcotic, some states limit its sale to pharmacists only while other states classify it as a prescription drug. Widespread abuse of dextromethorphan, especially by adolescents, may result in it soon becoming a pharmacist only available drug.[13]

Monograph ingredients
See table 4.3.

Warnings and precautions
Productive coughs associated with lower respiratory tract conditions that produce excessive phlegm or mucus require treatment by a physician. Chronic coughs associated with smoking, asthma, or emphysema should not be self-treated. Cough persisting for more than 7 days in adults or 5 days in children requires consultation with a physician.[12]

Codeine, dextromethorphan, and diphenhydramine may cause drowsiness, and codeine may cause constipation. Diphenhydramine is an antihistamine and its label must contain all the warning for antihistamines. Dextromethorphan should not be taken if individuals are taking a MAOI or for 2 weeks after stopping a MAOI, because high doses may cause increased central nervous system depression, hypertension, hyperpyrexia, and seizures.

Recommended dose
Dosages for antitussives are given in table 4.3.

Products
Diphenhydramine: (Benadryl and Theraflu MultiSymptom), dextromethorphan: (Robitussin Cough Gels, Triaminic Long Acting Cough, DayQuil Cough, Delsym, Robitussin Cough Gels, Robitussin DM (which also contains guaifenesin), Triaminic Long Acting Cough, and Vicks Formula 44 Dry Cough).

Peripheral or local acting antitussives

Mode of action
Vapors from aromatic compounds (camphor and menthol) are inhaled, reaching the mucous membranes of the mouth and nose. They produce a soothing effect on irritated membranes, thus reducing coughs caused by stimulation of peripheral nerves. Formulations include solutions for addition to vaporizers, devices to be plugged into electrical outlets, and devices for placement in showers. Ointments or patches may be applied to the chest and neck areas, and clothing should be left loose around the neck to allow the vapors to reach the nose and mouth.

Menthol as a lozenge formulation dissolves in the mouth, producing a local, soothing effect on the irritated oropharyngeal membranes to reduce coughs.

Monograph ingredients
See table 4.3.

Warnings and precautions
These compounds are for external use only and should not be taken by mouth, except for menthol lozenges. Liquid products should only be added to a vaporizer and not be left near an open flame. Ointments and chest rub products should not be used in the nose or under the nose, and should not be used in children under 2 years of age. There are several reports of severe respiratory effects from improper use of these products in infants and young children.

Recommended dose
Menthol cough drops, 5 to 10 mg, may be dissolved slowly in the mouth every 1 to 2 hours.

Products
Menthol lozenges (Hall's cough drops, N'ice, Ricola, Vick's cough drops). Menthol and camphor topical combinations (Vicks VapoRub Ointment and

TheraFlu Vapor Patch), plug-in devices (PediaCare Gentle Vapors, SudaCare Vapor-Plug Waterless Vaporizor, TheraFlu Flowing Vapors), or tablets to be placed in the shower (SudaCare Shower Soothers).

Expectorants

Drug category and indications for use
An expectorant helps to loosen phlegm, and makes coughs more productive.[14] Expectorants may relieve the congestion that frequently occurs with colds.

Monograph ingredients
Guaifenesin is the only FDA approved expectorant.

Mode of action
Expectorants may irritate the gastric mucosa, causing reflex stimulation of respiratory secretions, reducing the viscosity of bronchial secretions.[14]

Warning and precautions
Guaifenesin should not be taken for a chronic cough; a cough associated with asthma, chronic bronchitis, or emphysema; or a cough with excessive phlegm or mucus without consulting a physician.[14]

Recommended dose
Table 4.3 gives dosage for guaifenesin.

Products
Guaifenesin (Robitussin Chest Congestion, and Mucinex).

Combination cold products

The efficacy of antitussive and expectorant combinations in treating upper respiratory tract infections, especially when cough is present, appears to be a paradox. Meta-analysis reviews of randomized controlled studies of most combination cough and cold products in adults report only a slight positive effect compared with placebo.[15]

The FDA has declared that no OTC cough/cold product should be used for children under age 2 because of lack of efficacy and risk of adverse effects, and it is evaluating their use for children aged 2 to 11 years.[16] The Consumer Healthcare Products Association, which represents most OTC drug manufacturers, announced a voluntary relabeling of pediatric cough/cold products in October 2008. The new labels will instruct parents not to use cough/cold products in children under 4 years of age without the advise of a physician.[17]

Products
Robitussin DM, Vick's Formula 44 Custom Care Chesty Cough.

The number of products for cough/cold or flu treatment is somewhat overwhelming and popular products are listed in table 4.4. All the pharmacological classes of drug discussed in this chapter (antihistamines, decongestants, analgesics, antitussives, and expectorants) may be use alone or in multiple combinations.[10]

Table 4.4 Ingredients in popular cough/cold and flu products					
Product	Analgesic	Antihistamine	Antitussive	Decongestant	Expectorant
Alka Seltzer Plus cold	Yes	Yes		Yes	
Coricidin Maximum Strength Flu	Yes	Yes	Yes		
Dimetapp Cold & Cough		Yes	Yes	Yes	
Dimetapp Nighttime Flu	Yes	Yes	Yes	Yes	
Robitussin Cough & Cold			Yes	Yes	Yes
Robitussin Cough, Cold & Flu	Yes	Yes	Yes	Yes	
TheraFlu Cough & Cold		Yes	Yes	Yes	
Theraflu Warming Nighttime Severe Cold	Yes	Yes		Yes	
Triaminic Flu, Cough & Fever	Yes	Yes	Yes		
Triaminic Chest and Nasal Congestion				Yes	Yes
Tylenol Cold Multi-Symptom Severe	Yes		Yes	Yes	Yes
Tylenol Cough, Sore Throat Day	Yes		Yes		
Tylenol Plus Children's Flu	Yes	Yes	Yes	Yes	

Table 4.4 (continued)

Vicks Formula 44 Cough & Cold PM	Yes	Yes	Yes		
Vicks Formula 44 Congestion			Yes	Yes	
Vicks Formula 44 Chesty Cough			Yes		Yes
Vicks DayQuil Liquid	Yes		Yes	Yes	
Vicks NyQuil Liquid	Yes	Yes	Yes		
Vicks NyquilD	Yes	Yes	Yes	Yes	
Vicks Children's NyQuil		Yes	Yes		

Alternative therapy for colds and flu

Many consumers prefer the use of natural products such as rose hips, echinacea, or zinc for a cold because they have fewer adverse effects. These products do not have to prove safety or efficacy to the FDA before they appear in the marketplace.

Vitamin C

Rose hips are a natural source of vitamin C. There is no evidence that high doses of vitamin C prevent colds. Vitamin C in doses greater than 200 mg daily may reduce the severity of cold symptoms.[18]

Echinacea

Echinacea species (E. angustifolia, E. purpurea, and E. pallida) are dietary supplements promoted to prevent or treat colds. Lack of quality in the studies and uncertainty of the purity of the products hinders a true evaluation of these products. E. purpurea has been the most studied species and may have a mild effect in reducing duration and symptoms of colds. Individuals allergic to chrysanthemums may also be allergic to echinacea. Various parts of the plant have been used, but root extracts seem to be more effective.[19]

Zinc products

Zinc compounds as either dietary supplements or homeopathic products claim to bind to the ICAM-1 receptor present in nasal passages, preventing or reducing the risk of viral infection. A structured review of 11 published clinical trials demonstrated a slight positive effect in reducing cold symptoms, but a nearly equal number of studies showed no effect.[20] Limitations of most zinc studies include use of zinc salts other than zinc gluconate or zinc acetate, unknown concentrations of free zinc, and small numbers of study participants. The product's taste seems to be the most frequent complaint, and it may cause gastric upset. Many different flavors of lozenges are available to mask its astringent taste.

A recent randomized, double-blind, placebo-controlled clinical trial of individuals who began treatment within 24 hours of developing cold symptoms using zinc acetate lozenges (13.3 mg zinc) every 2 to 3 hours reported that both the duration (nearly 3 day reduction) and the severity of cold symptoms were significantly reduced. This study is important because it measured the plasma concentration of zinc and several of the inflammatory factors involved in producing cold symptoms, including ICAM-1 concentrations.[21]

Application of zinc intranasally has also produced positive results in reducing cold symptoms and duration, but there have been reports of individuals who have lost their sense of smell from this formulation.[22]

Products
Zinc gluconate (Cold-Eeze Lozenge, Zicam Lozenges contain zinc acetate and gluconate salts, Zicam Nasal Gel Swabs).

Oscillococcinum

Oscillococcinum is one of the most popular homeopathic flu products. It contains extracts from duck heart and liver, which are purported to be reservoir sites for the flu virus. There are relatively few placebo-controlled trials of this product despite the fact that it has been used for over a century. The most recent *Cochrane Review* notes that evidence of oscillococcinum's efficacy is lacking.[23]

Airborne

Airborne is a dietary supplement containing vitamins, herbs, and amino acids that is labeled as supporting the immune system. Several years ago, Oprah Winfrey and guests on her television show praised the ability of Airborne as a product that would prevent colds. This endorsement led to the product becoming a huge success. Closer examination of the product's ingredients and lack of supportive studies have seen its popularity decline. The product originally claimed to prevent and cure colds, which, as a dietary supplement, it cannot do. The company agreed to a $23.3 million settlement with refunds to go to buyers.[24]

The product contains vitamins A, C, E, and riboflavin, several minerals, amino acids, and echinacea. A single tablet contains 230 mg sodium and the recommended dose of three tablets daily would greatly exceed the amount of sodium permitted for individuals who are on a sodium-restricted diet. There is no evidence of its effectiveness.

Asthma

Asthma is a lower respiratory system condition characterized by impaired airflow in the bronchial tubes and lungs. The bronchi are hyper-responsive to certain stimuli, producing an inflammatory response causing constriction and narrowing of the airways accompanied by excessive secretions. The respiratory system responds to these symptoms by increasing its release of epinephrine, a neurotransmitter. Epinephrine activates specific receptors, beta-2-adrenoceptors, in the sympathetic nervous system and these cause the bronchi to dilate to make breathing easier.

Epinephrine

Drug category and indications for use
OTC bronchodilating drugs are used to provide symptomatic relief of wheezing and shortness of breath only if the patient has been diagnosed by a physician as having asthma.[25]

Mode of action
Exogenous epinephrine binds to the beta-2-adrenoceptors in the bronchi in the same manner as endogenously produced epinephrine, causing bronchodilatation and improving breathing.

Monograph ingredients
Epinephrine and its salts are available for inhalation using hand-held nebulizers or metered-dose inhalers.[25]

Warnings and precautions
Epinephrine products should not be used by those with heart disease, high blood pressure, thyroid disease, diabetes, or difficulty in urinating because of an enlarged prostate unless directed by a physician. They also should not be used by anyone taking a prescription drug for asthma, high blood pressure, or depression (MAOIs). They may cause nervousness, tremors, insomnia, nausea, rapid heart beat, or loss of appetite.[25] The products should not be used if cloudy or discolored. Epinephrine products should not be used in children under 4 years of age; for children 4 years or older, one inhalation is used, repeated if necessary after a wait of 1 minute; the inhaler should not be used again for at least 3 hours and a physician should be consulted if symptoms are not relieved. For adults, use should not continue if symptoms are not relieved in 20 minutes or if they become worse and a physician should be consulted.

Recommended dose
Dosages for broncholdilators are listed in table 4.3.

Products
Epinephrine (micro Nephrin for nebulizers and Primatene Mist).

Oral inhalers may be removed from the OTC market because chloro-fluorocarbon propellants currently in these products must be replaced under regulations from the Environmental Protection Agency. Manufacturers would have to reformulate their products and apply to the FDA for approval, a very costly process.

Pharmacists should counsel and encourage patients who purchase OTC bronchodilators that they should consult a physician. The OTC products have limited use because optimum treatment for asthma patients requires prescription corticosteroids, beta-2 sympathomimetics, or leukotriene receptor antagonist drugs.

Ephedrine

Mode of action
Ephedrine is a drug that mimics the action of epinephrine by binding to the beta-2-adrenoceptors in the lungs, causing bronchodilatation. It is effective as an oral drug, in contrast to epinephrine, which is destroyed in the stomach and must be inhaled.

Monograph ingredients
Ephedrine and its salts.

Warnings and precautions
Ephedrine should not be used in children under 12 years of age. Use should not be continued if symptoms are not relieved in 1 hour or become worse and a physician should be consulted immediately.

Recommended dose
Dosage is given in table 4.3.

Products
Ephedrine (Bronkaid Dual Action Formula and Primatene).

Case study exercises

Case 1 A mother asks the pharmacist to recommend an antihistamine for her 4-year-old child who is allergic to grass and tree pollens.
Several recommendations are possible, including sodium cromolyn, but a loratadine tablet that dissolves on the tongue or a liquid

formulation is a good choice for this child. Sodium cromolyn must be used 1 to 2 weeks before exposure to the allergen for maximum benefit, and first-generation antihistamines may cause to much drowsiness.

Case 2 A 68-year-old man asks the pharmacist to recommend an antihistamine because he is allergic to grasses. His prescription record contains Flomax for a prostate problem.
Cromolyn sodium would have no effect on his benign prostatic hyperplasia (BPH); although it may not be as effective as antihistamine, it will prevent or reduce his symptoms if used prophylactically according to the directions. Cetirizine and loratadine are the only OTC antihistamines that do not contain BPH warnings and could be used. However, the individual is over 65 and should consult his physician before using cetirizine.

Case 3 GH, 15-year-old female, experiences nasal congestion and mild rhinitis when she visits her friend who has a cat. She asks the pharmacist for Sudafed.
Because GH is under 18, the pharmacist recommends Sudafed PE, which will help to reduce the nasal congestions and rhinitis. Sudafed is pseudoephedrine and may only be sold to individuals 18 years of age or older. However, an antihistamine such as loratadine taken approximately 30 minutes before going to her friend's house would be more effective by preventing the histamine release that causes her symptoms. The best recommendation is to avoid the cat and the areas that it frequents.

Case 4 RT asks the pharmacist to recommend a sleeping tablet. He tells the pharmacist that he began using Sinex spray approximately 3 weeks ago because he gets nasal congestion during the evenings, and several days later he began having sleeping problems.
The pharmacist explains that the phenylephrine in the Sinex is probably the cause of his problem and he should limit or stop using Sinex before bedtime. No sedative is needed. The pharmacist advises RT to limit his use of Sinex because excess use (more than 3 days in the labeling) increases the risk of developing rebound congestion. The pharmacist recommends trying Breathe Right Strips. If RT continues to have problems sleeping, he could try using an OTC sedative or he should consult his physician.

Case 5 A mother of a 3-year-old child asks the pharmacist for advice in treating her child who has a cough from a cold.

The use of a steam vaporizer with camphor or menthol is the safest choice because of lack of adverse effects. If the mother is concerned about the child potentially getting burned by the heated water, a cool mist humidifier or an ultrasonic humidifier without aromatic vapors may be used. A plug-in vaporizer product is another alternative. The FDA currently does not recommend OTC cough/cold products for children under 4 years of age unless a physician has been consulted.

References

1. Cold, cough, allergy, bronchodilator, and antiasthmatic drug products for over-the-counter human use; final monograph for OTC antihistamine drug products; final rule. *Fed Regist* 1992; 57: 58356–58376.
2. Abbas AK. Diseases of immunity. In: Kumar V, Abbas AK, Fausto N, eds. *Robbins and Cotran: Pathologic Basis of Disease*, 7th edn. Philadelphia, PA: Elsevier Saunders, 2005: 193–267.
3. Rosenfeld RM.Clinical practice guideline on adult sinusitis. *Otolaryngol Head Neck Surg* 2007; 137: 365–377.
4. Zyrtec. www.Zyrtec.com (accessed September 29, 2008).
5. Claritin. www.Claritin.com (accessed September 29, 2008).
6. www.NasalCrom.com (accessed September 29, 2008).
7. Cold, cough, allergy, bronchodilator, and antiasthmatic drug products for over-the-counter human use; final monograph for OTC nasal decongestant drug products; final rule. *Fed Regist* 1994; 59: 43386–43412.
8. Legal requirements for the sale and purchase of drug products containing pseudoephedrine, ephedrine, and phenylpropanolamine. www.fda.gov/cder/news/methamaphetamine.htm (accessed September 10, 2008).
9. Kirkness JP *et al.* Nasal airflow dynamics; mechanisms and responses with an external nasal dilator strip. *Eur Respir J* 2000; 15: 929–936.
10. Cold, cough, allergy, bronchodilator, and antiasthmatic drug products for over-the-counter human use; final monograph for combination drug products. Final Rule. *Fed Regist* 2002; 67: 78158–78172.
11. Bolser DC. Cough suppressant and pharmacologic protussive therapy ACCP Evidenced-based clinical practice guidelines. Chest. 2006; 129(1Suppl):238S–249S.
12. Cold, cough, allergy, bronchodilator, and antiasthmatic drug products for over-the-counter human use; final monograph for OTC antitussive drug products; Final Rule. *Fed Regist* 1987; 52: 30042–30057.
13. *The National Survey on Drug Use and Health Report*. January 2008. http://oas.samhsa.gov/2k8/cough/cough.htm (accessed March 17, 2008).
14. Cold, cough, allergy, bronchodilator, and antiasthmatic drug products for over-the-counter human use; Expectorant drug products for over-the-counter human use; final monograph; final rule. *Fed Regist* 1989; 54: 8494–8509.
15. Smith SM *et al.* OTC medications for acute cough in children and adults in ambulatory settings. *Cochrane Database Syst Rev* 2008 (1): CD001831.
16. FDA News. *FDA Releases Recommendations Regarding Use of OTC Cough and Cold Products.* www.fda.gov/bbs/topics/NEWS/2008/NEW01778.html (accessed January 18, 2008).
17. *Transcript of Media Briefing on Pediatric Over-the-Counter Nonprescription Cough and Cold Products.* www.fda.gov/bbs/transcripts/2008/otc100708.pdf (accessed October 28, 2008).

18. Douglas RM. Vitamin C for preventing and treating the common cold. *Cochrane Database Syst Rev* 2007; (3): CD000980.
19. Shah S *et al*. Evaluation of Echinacea for the prevention and treatment of the common cold: a meta-analysis. *Lancet Infect Dis* 2007; 7: 473–480.
20. Caruso TJ *et al*. Treatment of naturally acquired common colds with zinc: a structured review. *Clin Infect Dis* 2007; 45: 569–574.
21. Prasad AS *et al*. Duration and severity of symptoms and levels of plasma interleuleukin-1 receptor antagonist, soluble tumor necrosis factor receptor, and adhesion molecules in patients with common cold treated with zinc acetate. *J Infect Dis* 2008; 197: 795–802.
22. Hirt M *et al*. Zinc nasal gel for treatment of common cold symptoms: a double-blind, placebo-controlled trial. *Ear Nose Throat J* 2000; 79: 778–782.
23. Vickers A, Smith C. Homoeopathic oscillicoccinum for preventing and treating influenza and influenza-like syndromes. *Cochrane Database Syst Rev* 2006; (3): CD001957.
24. *Maker of Airborne will pay refunds for product that was marketed as a cold preventative.* www.webMD.com/cold-and-flu/news/20080304/coldremedy-airborne-settles-lawsuit?page=2 (accessed March 14, 2009).
25. Cold, cough, allergy, bronchodilator, and antiasthmatic drug products for over-the-counter human use; final monograph for OTC bronchodilator drug products; final rule. *Fed Regist* 1986; 51: 35326–35340.

5

Central nervous system (including peripheral analgesics)

This chapter discusses oral analgesic/antipyretic drugs, sedatives, and stimulants. Sedative and stimulant drugs act directly on receptors in various parts of the brain while OTC internal analgesics first react in the periphery to inhibit the synthesis of a series of compounds known as prostaglandins. All of the OTC analgesics have an antipyretic effect, reducing an elevated body temperature by acting on the hypothalamus in the brain. The brain and spinal cord make up the central nervous system (CNS).

Many of the effects of prostaglandins are produced locally in tissues, but some of their analgesic effects may be mediated by stimulating neurons in the peripheral nervous system. Nerves from the peripheral nervous system propagate signals to the spinal cord that reach the brain via afferent nerve pathways. Transmission of nerve impulses from the brain and spinal cord to the peripheral tissues occurs via efferent nerve fibers.

Oral OTC analgesic drugs do not identify the cause of pain nor do they correct it; they merely prevent or relieve mild to moderate pain. External analgesics are drugs applied topically to the skin or mucous membranes to block or prevent transmission from the peripheral nervous system. External OTC analgesics are discussed separately Chapters 7 (topical OTC oral cavity products) and 8 (topical OTC drugs for dermatological conditions).

OTC analgesics include acetaminophen and several drugs known as nonsteroidal anti-inflammatory drugs (NSAIDs), which include aspirin, other salicylate drugs, ibuprofen, naproxen sodium, and ketoprofen. All of the drugs produce analgesic and antipyretic effects, but acetaminophen has little to no effect on inflammation.

The FDA has approved caffeine as a monograph analgesic adjuvant. An adjuvant is a drug that does not have any analgesic activity but if combined with an approved analgesic provides greater pain relief than the analgesic by itself.[1]

Acetaminophen, aspirin, and ibuprofen may be used for all types of headache including migraine headache. Manufacturers of products labeled exclusively for migraine pain obtained FDA approval by submitting additional data. Directions for use of these products differs from their use as ordinary analgesic/antipyretic products.[2]

Oral analgesics

Acetaminophen

Acetaminophen is one of the most widely used analgesics in the USA. It is used OTC for all age groups over the age of 2 years and is prescribed by healthcare professionals for those under 2 years of age. It is the analgesic least likely to cause GI symptoms, gastric irritation, GI bleeding, and ulcers, and it does not affect blood platelets.

Acetaminophen is metabolized by the liver and is associated with liver toxicity and death. This risk is increased if the use of acetaminophen involves high daily doses, a long period of use, or the ingestion of three or more alcohol beverages per day. Accidental ingestions by children or adults require immediate treatment, even if there are no immediate symptoms of toxicity.

Drug category and indications for use
Acetaminophen is an analgesic and antipyretic. It may be used to reduce fevers and provide temporary relief for minor aches and pains caused by the common cold, sore throat, toothache, headache, muscular aches and pain, premenstrual and menstrual cramps (dysmenorrhea), and pain associated with arthritis.[1]

Monograph ingredient
Acetaminophen.

Mode of action
Acetaminophen is a weak inhibitor of prostaglandin synthesis in the periphery but has a more pronounced effect in the brain; its full mechanism of action remains uncertain. It has no true anti-inflammatory activity as NSAIDs have, but it is recommended as a primary drug for relieving mild to moderate arthritic pain. Two basic reasons for its use are that much of the pain associated with osteoarthritis is not from an inflammatory process and its safety profile for those over the age of 60 years is much better than that of the NSAIDs.[3]

Warnings and precautions
Adults and children over 12 years of age should not exceed the recommended dose of 4 g per 24 hours because severe liver damage may occur at higher dosage. Acetaminophen should not be used without consulting a physician if

an individual has liver disease. If the individual consumes three or more alcoholic drinks every day, a physician should be consulted before taking this product. OTC acetaminophen should not be used with any other drugs, prescription or nonprescription, containing acetaminophen. A physician or pharmacist should be consulted by anyone unsure of the content of other drugs they are taking.[4,5]

Acetaminophen should not be used for more than 10 days for temporary relief of pain and for not more than 3 days if used for fever. If fever occurs or swelling or redness occurs at the site of pain, a physician should be consulted. Products labeled for sore throat pain are limited to 2 days of use. If the pain worsens or a fever develops, a physician should be consulted.[1,5,6]

Children under 12 years of age should not take more than five doses of acetaminophen in a 24 hour period because it could cause severe liver damage. The drug should not be used without consulting a physician if the child has liver damage or if the child is taking any other product that contains acetaminophen. If the caregiver is unsure of the content of other drugs the child is taking, a physician or pharmacist should be consulted.

Acetaminophen products for children 2 to 12 years of age should not be labeled for use of muscle aches and pains, premenstrual or menstrual cramps, or arthritis.[5,6]

The FDA issued a final monograph for labeling of all internal analgesics on April 29, 2009. Even though acetaminophen does not affect blood platelets, all acetaminophen products must contain a warning by April 2010 that a physician or pharmacist should be consulted if the individual is taking warfarin.[6] Maximum doses of acetaminophen taken for 1 week or more increase the anticoagulant effect of warfarin by influencing its pharmacokinetics.[7]

NOTE: All these warnings about acetaminophen are required to be on the product's label when acetaminophen is combined in cough/cold products, sinus pain relief products, premenstrual and menstrual pain relief products, or sedative products.[5,6]

In June 2009, an FDA Advisory Committee recommended stronger warnings or perhaps removal of acetaminophen from many combination prescription products because of accidental overdoses.[7] These recommendations may extend to nonprescription products in the future, especially allergy/cough/cold products. Such a change would affect many products on the market and may result in formulation changes.

Recommended dose
Adults and children over 12 may take one or two 325 mg (regular strength) or 500 mg tablets (extra strength) every 4 to 6 hours, but should not exceed 4000 mg in 24 hours; sustained release acetaminophen is available as 650 mg tablets and one to two tablets may be taken every 8 hours but must be swallowed, not chewed or crushed.[5,6]

Table 5.1 Recommended doses of acetaminophen syrup or suspension (160 mg per teaspoon (tsp) or 5 mL) for children 2–12 years of age

Weight (lbs)	Weight (kg)	Age (years)	Oral dose[a]
Under 24	Under 11	Under 2	Consult doctor
24–35	11–16	2–3	1 tsp or 5 mL (160 mg)
36–47	16.3–21.3	4–5	1.5 tsp or 7.5 mL (240 mg)
48–59	21.8–26.8	6–8	2 tsp or 10 mL (320 mg)
60–71	27.2–32.2	8–10	2.5 tsp or 12.5 mL (400 mg)
72–95	32.7–43.2	11–12	3 tsp or 15 mL (480 mg)

[a]Doses should be measured only with the measuring device enclosed in the package.

The recommended doses of acetaminophen syrup or suspension for children between the ages of 2 and 12 years are given in table 5.1 and for concentrated infant acetaminophen drops in table 5.2.

Concentrated infants drops contain more acetaminophen per milliliter than do syrup or suspension formulations and should only be measured with the dropper that is packaged with the container. Failure to use the appropriate measuring device may result in improper doses and is a frequent cause of overdoses when the concentrated infant drops are used.

Products

Tylenol Regular Strength, Tylenol Extra Strength, Tylenol 8 hour, Tylenol Arthritis, Feverall Suppositories, and Panadol.

NOTE: Tylenol 8 hour may be used in children over 12 years of age and Tylenol Arthritis may be use in individuals over 18 years of age. Both contain the same formula of sustained release acetaminophen, but arthritis products may not be labeled for use in individuals under 18 years of age. Arthritis that occurs in a child or adolescent requires physician treatment, not self-care.

Table 5.2 Recommended doses for concentrated acetaminophen infant drops (concentration, 80 mg in 0.8 mL; 1 dropperful is 0.8 mL)

Weight (lbs)	Weight (kg)	Age (years)	Dose
Under 24	Under 11	Under 2	Consult doctor
24–35	11–16	2–3	1.6 mL (use two dropperful doses of 0.8 mL) (160 mg)

Nonsteroidal anti-inflammatory analgesic/antipyretic drugs

Monograph drugs

Aspirin (acetylsalicylic acid), carbaspirin calcium, choline salicylate, magnesium salicylate, sodium salicylate, ibuprofen, naproxen sodium, and ketoprofen are all classified as NSAIDs.

Drug category and indications for use

NSAIDs may be used to reduce fever and provide temporary relief for minor aches and pains caused by the common cold, sore throat, headache, muscular aches and pain, backache, premenstrual and menstrual cramps (dysmenorrhea), and pain associated with arthritis.[1,5,6]

Low-dose aspirin (81 mg per day) may be recommended by a physician to prevent the aggregation of blood platelets to reduce the risk of heart attacks and strokes in certain individuals.

Mode of action

Aspirin and the other salicylates combine with cyclo-oxygenase enzymes (COX-1 and COX-2), which are responsible for the first step in the formation of prostaglandins and thromboxanes from arachidonic acid in the periphery. Prostaglandins are produced in the inflammatory response and are involved in the production of pain, especially pain associated with headache and premenstrual and menstrual pain. The anti-inflammatory effect of aspirin and salicylates derives from their ability to inhibiting prostaglandin synthesis. Consequently, they are known as nonsteroidal anti-inflammatory drugs, NSAIDs.[3]

Prostaglandin E_2 (PGE$_2$) produced in the periphery increases cyclic adenosine monophosphate (cyclic AMP), which causes the hypothalamus to increase body temperature. Aspirin and the other NSAIDs inhibit PGE$_2$ synthesis, thus having an antipyretic effect.[3]

Prostaglandin H_2 is converted to thromboxanes, which are involved in platelet aggregation to stop bleeding. Because aspirin, but not other salicylates, binds irreversibly to the acetyl site of COX-1, it is used for its anticoagulant activity in individuals who are at risk for heart attacks and strokes that are caused by blood clots. Individuals should consult their physician before using aspirin for these cardiovascular uses.[1,3,5–8]

Aspirin, carbaspirin calcium, choline salicylate, magnesium salicylate, sodium salicylate, and ibuprofen administered in recommended doses have the same efficacy as analgesics and antipyretics.[1,5]

Warnings and precautions

Individuals allergic to aspirin or any other pain or fever relief drug should not take the drug as they may experience hives, asthma (wheezing), facial swelling, or shock. The drug should be stopped immediately if any of these symptoms occur and a physician should be contacted.[1,5,6]

Children and teenagers should not use this drug if they have recovered, or are recovering, from flu or chickenpox because they may develop Reye's syndrome, a serious condition associated with the use of aspirin and salicylates.[5,6,9] Reye's syndrome occurs usually after a viral infection such as chickenpox or flu. Symptoms include persistent vomiting, fatigue, and confusion, and the syndrome may progress to convulsions, unconsciousness, and death. There is an increase in intracranial pressure and increased fatty deposits in the liver and other organs. Immediate treatment minimizes the residual effects of this condition.[10]

All NSAIDs may cause stomach bleeding and the risk of this event is greater if individuals are over 60 years of age, have bleeding problems, peptic ulcer disease, diabetes, gout, or arthritis, or if the individual is taking an anticoagulant drug (blood thinner), steroids, or any other drugs containing NSAIDs. Consuming three or more alcoholic beverages a day, taking more than the recommended dose, or taking the drug for a longer period of time than recommended increases the risk of bleeding.[5,6]

The appearance of blood or occult blood in any vomit or stool may indicate stomach bleeding, and a physician should be consulted immediately. If an individual experiences stomach pain or ringing in the ears, a physician should be consulted.[5,6]

If NSAIDs do not relieve pain within 10 days, or fever within 3 days, a physician should be consulted. If the symptoms worsen or redness develops in the area of the pain, a physician should be consulted. If the product is labeled for sore throat pain, its use should be limited to 2 days.[1,5,6]

NSAIDs should not be used during the last 3 months of pregnancy unless directed by a physician because it may cause problems for the unborn child and complications during delivery.[1,5]

Aspirin should not be used to reduce the risk of a heart attack unless advised to do so by a physician.[5]

If a magnesium salicylate product has more than 50 milliequivalents of magnesium in the recommended daily dose, it should not be used by individuals with kidney disease without consulting a physician.[1]

If individuals have diabetes, high blood pressure, kidney disease or take a diuretic drug, a physician should be consulted before using any NSAID. NSAIDs may inhibit prostaglandins that produce vasodilatation of blood vessels in the kidney, resulting in vasoconstriction and causing an increase in blood pressure, further compromising kidney function in individuals who have kidney disease.[6,11,12]

There are two special warnings for ibuprofen in addition to all the other NSAIDs warnings.

Special ibuprofen warning for concomitant use with low-dose aspirin (81 mg). There is competitive action between ibuprofen and aspirin for the acetyl-binding site of cyclo-oxygenase when both drugs are administered together. Since this is the site where aspirin acts to prevent platelet aggregation for its cardiovascular effect, its effectiveness will be reduced. If an individual uses both drugs, aspirin should be administered 8 hours after ibuprofen.[13] There is little evidence that naproxen sodium and ketoprofen might have the same effect.

Special ibuprofen warning for migraine headache use. Individuals should not use ibuprofen for a migraine headache if a physician has never diagnosed their problem as a migraine headache. If the headache differs from previous migraine headaches, is the worst headache of their life, is accompanied by a fever and stiff neck, or has occurred after a head injury, a physician should be consulted. If the headache is caused by bending, coughing, or exertion, occurs daily, or is accompanied by vomiting, a physician should be consulted before using ibuprofen. Ibuprofen is not recommended for treating migraine headaches in individuals under 18 years of age unless a recommendation was made by a physician.[14]

Recommended dose

Aspirin for pain or fever relief. Adults and children over 12 years of age may take two tablets of either 325 mg (regular strength) or 500 mg (extra strength) aspirin per dose every 4 to 6 hours, not exceeding 12 tablets within 24 hours. Although the monograph permits aspirin use in children under 12 years of age, most healthcare professionals do not recommend its use; acetaminophen is the preferred drug in children under 12 years of age.[1,6]

Aspirin for reduction of cardiovascular risk. The dose of aspirin recommended is 81 mg per day for most individuals (a 'baby' aspirin), but this use should be discussed with a physician. Doses higher than 81 mg (325 to 500 mg) may be recommended by a physician for certain individuals.

Salicylate drugs. Dose recommendations are given in table 5.3.

Table 5.3 Recommended adult doses of analgesic/antipyretic salicylate drugs (maximum 4 times a day)

Drug	Adult dose (mg)
Aspirin	325–1000
Carbaspirin calcium	414–828
Choline salicylate	435–870
Sodium salicylate	250–650
Magnesium salicylate	325–650

Table 5.4 Recommended doses of ibuprofen for children under 12 years of age (100 mg in 1 teaspoon (tsp) or 5 milliliters (mL).

Weight (lbs)	Weight (kg)	Age (years)	Dose
Under 24	Under 11	Under 2	Consult doctor
24–35	11–16	2–3	1 tsp or 5 mL (100 mg)
36–47	16.3–21.3	4–5	1.5 tsp or 7.5 mL (150 mg)
48–59	21.8–26.8	6–8	2 tsp or 10 mL (200 mg)
60–71	27.2–32.2	9–10	2.5 tsp or 12.5 mL (250 mg)
72–95	32.7–43.2	11–12	3 tsp or 15 mL (300 mg)

Ibuprofen. Dose recommendation for adults and children over 12 years of age is 200 to 400 mg per dose up to four times a day. Children's ibuprofen has a longer duration of action than acetaminophen and is given every 6 to 8 hours. Table 5.4 has the recommended doses for children aged between 2 and 12 years and table 5.5 for concentrated ibuprofen infants drops.

Products

Aspirin (Bayer Aspirin, Ascriptin, Anacin (contains caffeine as an adjuvant), Bufferin, and Ecotrin (enteric coated aspirin), choline salicylate (Arthropan is a liquid formulation), magnesium salicylate (Mobigesic, Backache Maximum Strength, Extra Strength Doan's, and Momentum Muscular Backache). NOTE: There is no evidence that any of these products are more effective in treating backache pain than any other aspirin or salicylate product, despite the name of specific products.

Low-dose aspirin (81 mg) products: Bayer Low Dose 'Baby' Aspirin, St. Joseph Adult Low Strength Aspirin.

Ibuprofen (Advil, Advil Infants' Concentrated Drops, Advil Children's Suspension, Advil Migraine, and Motrin IB, Junior Strength Motrin, Concentrated Motrin Children's Drops).

Table 5.5 Recommended doses for concentrated ibuprofen infant drops (50 mg in 1.25 mL; special measuring device included in package)

Weight (lbs)	Weight (kg)	Age (months)	Dose
		Under 6	Consult doctor
12–17	5.5–7.7	6–11	1.25 mL (50 mg)
18–23	8.2–10.5	12–23	1.875 mL (75 mg)

Rx–OTC switched NSAIDs

Drug category and indications for use
NSAIDs may be used to reduce fevers and provide temporary relief for minor aches and pains caused by the common cold, sore throat, toothache, headache, muscular aches and pain, backache, premenstrual and menstrual cramps (dysmenorrhea), and pain associated with arthritis.

OTC NSAIDs
Ibuprofen, naproxen sodium and ketoprofen are available as analgesic/antipyretic drugs because manufacturers submitted abbreviated new drug applications. These drugs are available as prescription products but in doses that are higher than those in OTC products. The FDA included ibuprofen in the OTC Internal Analgesic Monograph in 2002.[15]

Mode of action
NSAIDs inhibit the synthesis of prostaglandins in peripheral tissues and act in the hypothalamus to reduce a fever in the same manner as aspirin. However, NSAIDs competively inhibit cyclo-oxygenase in a reversible manner. These NSAIDs cause somewhat less gastric irritation and bleeding than aspirin but require the same warnings.[5,6]

Warnings and precautions
If individuals are allergic to ibuprofen, naproxen sodium, ketoprofen, or aspirin, or any other analgesic medication, they should not take theses product, because they may cause hives, asthma (wheezing), or facial swelling. The drug should be stopped immediately if any of these symptoms occur and a physician contacted.

These products may cause stomach bleeding and the risk of this event is greater if individuals are over 60 years of age, have bleeding problems or peptic ulcer disease, take an anticoagulant drug (blood thinner), take steroids, take any other drugs containing NSAIDs (either OTC or prescription), drink three or more alcoholic beverages a day, take more than the recommended dose, or take the drug for a longer period of time than recommended. A physician or pharmacist should be consulted when taking other drugs if individuals do not know the content of other medications.[5,6]

If blood appears in any vomiting or the stools have blood or are very black, this may indicate stomach bleeding, and a physician should be consulted immediately. If an individual experiences stomach pain or ringing in the ears, a physician should be consulted.

If the product does not relieving pain within 10 days, or fever within 3 days, a physician should be consulted. If the symptoms worsen or redness develops in the area of the pain, a physician should be consulted. If the product is labeled for sore throat pain, its use should be limited to 2 days.[1,5]

A physician should be consulted before using these products if the individual has diabetes, high blood pressure, liver cirrhosis, or kidney disease.[6]

These drugs should not be used during the last 3 months of pregnancy unless told to do so by a physician, because they may cause problems for the unborn child and complications during delivery.[1,5]

Recommended dose

Naproxen sodium. Individuals between the ages of 12 and 65 years of age may take 220 mg (one tablet) every 8 to 12 hours and no more than three tablets within 24 hours. Adults over 60 years of age should take 220 mg (one tablet) every 12 hours. Children under 12 years of age should only take naproxen sodium if recommended by a physician.[16]

Ketoprofen. Adults and children over 16 years of age may take 12.5 mg ketoprofen every 8 hours. Children under 16 years of age should only take ketoprofen if recommended by a physician.

Products

Naproxen sodium (Aleve), ketoprofen (marketed as Orudis KT but discontinued by the manufacturer).

Analgesic combinations

The only permitted combination of analgesic drugs is acetaminophen and aspirin.[1]

Monograph ingredients

Acetaminophen and aspirin may be combined in a single product. The indications for use of each drug are the same, and the warnings and precautions for each drug must appear on the label. The combination drug may not be labeled for cardiovascular use even though it contains aspirin.

Special warnings for Excedrin Migraine

Individuals should not use Excedrin Migraine for a migraine headache if a physician has never diagnosed their problem as a migraine headache. If this headache is different from previous migraine headaches, is the worst headache of their life, is accompanied by a fever and stiff neck, or has occurred after a head injury, a physician should be consulted. If the headache is caused by bending, coughing or exertion, occurs daily, or is accompanied by vomiting, a physician should be consulted before using this product. Individuals under 18 years of age should not use this product for a migraine headache unless a recommendation has been made by their physician.[16] These warnings are in addition to all other acetaminophen and aspirin warnings that must appear on the label.

Products

Excedrin Extra Strength, Excedrin Migraine, Goody's Headache Powders, Vanquish.

Excedrin Extra Strength and Excedrin Migraine contain exactly the same drugs, acetaminophen (250 mg), aspirin (250 mg) and caffeine (65 mg), but the indications for use and labeled warnings are different. Excedrin Migraine has only one indication, migraine headache, and is labeled for use by individuals over 18 years of age; it has no other intended analgesic or antipyretic use.[17] Both drugs must have a warning for caffeine that states that the recommended dose of this product has caffeine that is about equal to a cup of coffee. Limit intake of caffeine from other sources to avoid nervousness, irritability, increased heart rate, and insomnia that occurs from too much caffeine.[17]

Sedatives

Sleep is a dynamic process divided into two components, rapid eye movement (REM) and nonrapid eye movement (NREM), which are easily distinguished by electrophysiological patterns that can be measured using electroencephalography (EEG) and electrooculography (EOG). These patterns vary depending on age of the individual and may be altered by environmental conditions and/or by an individual's mood, emotional state, drug therapy, or disease state.

NREM sleep has four stages, each stage being considered to be a deeper form of sleep. Stage 1 is the transition to sleep phase or the period for onset of sleep. Stage 2 is an intermediate stage, which accounts for approximately 40 to 50% of sleep. Stages 3 and 4 are deep sleep stages where EEG measurements show slow-moving waves. Stages 3 and 4 account for approximately 20% of sleep time and are primarily responsible for the restorative nature of sleep, described by individuals as feeling more alert and energetic after sleep. Stage 4 sleep becomes shorter in duration as people age and is partly responsible for the early awakening experienced by elderly individuals.[18]

REM sleep patterns are more complex and less predictable than NREM patterns and are associated with dreams. There is complete relaxation of voluntary muscles during NREM sleep, and memory enforcement occurs during this time. As the amount of REM sleep increases during the night, there is a decrease in stages 3 and 4 of NREM sleep. Individuals usually progress through four or five cycles of sleep (NREM and REM) during the night, with each cycle lasting approximately 90 to 120 minutes.[18]

Sleep is not a period where all biological systems shift into a lower activity level for a type of rest up or power up for the next day. Many important activities occur during sleep, for example growth hormone and cortisol (hydrocortisone) are secreted during sleep.

Insomnia is a general term that describes sleep disorders, and the most common complaint by healthy individuals is that of not being able to fall asleep readily, a sleep induction problem. The FDA's definition of an OTC sedative or nighttime sleep-aid is an agent that helps individuals who have occasional difficulty in falling asleep.[12] However, sleep is affected by external and internal factors, and individuals as well as pharmacists should have an understanding of the sleep process to determine when self-care may be appropriate.

The internal or intrinsic control for sleep is the suprachiasmatic nucleus (SCN) in the hypothalamus of the brain, which increases its neuronal signals as evening approaches (diminishing light), stimulating the pineal gland to secrete the hormone melatonin. Melatonin levels increase until about 2 to 4 a.m. and begin to diminish as dawn approaches. Estrogen and progesterone levels in the brain also affect the SCN and are probably responsible for the fact the women have a higher incidence of insomnia during menstruation and menopause. Postpartum women also have more problems with insomnia.[18]

The normal circadian rhythm in humans is slightly more than 24 hours. However, external cues, primarily light and darkness and the daily activities of individuals, entrain the daily rhythm to a 24 hour pattern and keep it at 24 hours. Light, either sunlight or bright artificial light, enters through the eyes, activating neural pathways to the brain to promote wakefulness. Physical activity, social interactions, and a busy or noisy environment also promote wakefulness.

Individuals who experience occasional insomnia should be evaluated for external causes of the problem before drug therapy is initiated. Behaviors that enhance readiness for sleep in individuals include no napping during the day, tapering down physical activity at the end of the day, having a regular pattern of activity to prepare for sleep, having a regular time to go to sleep, reducing distracting environmental factors such as too much light or noise, controlling the temperature so it is not too hot or too cold, avoiding stimulating drugs (caffeine in any form, pseudoephedrine or phenylephrine in allergy or cough/cold medications) in the evening, avoiding alcohol, and avoiding smoking. If these practices do not solve the individual's insomnia, OTC sedative or dietary supplements may help to alleviate the problem.

Common causes of sleep problems include shift work, jet travel, anxiety and stressful situations, and medical conditions such as asthma, chronic obstructive pulmonary disease, depression, sleep apnea, pain, dementia, and rhinitis, among others. Treatment of the medical condition by a physician should be the first attempt at solving sleep problems associated with medical problems.

Shift workers and travelers who going through numerous time zones have difficulties because each of these situations imposes new cues on the body's internal circadian rhythm. Melatonin has some positive effects in these situations, but prescription drugs are usually more effective. If shift work is a long-term employment situation, altering circadian rhythm by entrainment methods using light therapy and behavior modification may be successful.

Individuals who suffer from lack of sleep often complain of tiredness, fatigue, lack of mental alertness, decreased motor skill, lack of concentration, and irritability. Frequently, individuals try to compensate for these effects by using stimulant drugs.

OTC drugs

Monograph drug: diphenhydramine

Drug category and indications for use
Nighttime sleep-aid or sedative relieves occasional sleeplessness for individuals who have difficulty in falling asleep.[19]

Mode of action
Antihistamines classified as first generation or sedating antihistamines produce their effect by acting in the CNS.

Warnings and precautions
If diphenhydramine does not provide relief of sleeplessness within 2 weeks, a physician should be consulted because a more serious condition may be the problem. If an individual has asthma, glaucoma, emphysema, chronic pulmonary disease, shortness of breath, or difficulty in urinating because of an enlarged prostate, a physician should be consulted. Alcoholic beverages should not be consumed while taking diphenhydramine. If an individual is taking other sedatives or tranquilizers, a physician should be consulted before using this drug.[19]

Recommended dose
Adults and children over 12 years of age may take a single dose of 50 mg of diphenhydramine 30 minutes before bedtime. This product should not be used if any other product containing diphenhydramine is being used, even if it is for topical use.[20]

NOTE: Diphenhydramine in used in many oral products for allergies, sinus congestion, cough/colds, and itching, as well as topical products for insect bites and itching. There are many reports of toxicity because of the use of several products containing diphenhydramine.[20]

Products
Diphenhydramine: (Benadryl, Nytol, Simply Sleep, Sominex, Unisom Sleep Gels, and Unisom Sleep Melts).

Rx–OTC switched drug: doxylamine

Doxylamine is an approved antihistamine with sedative actions similar to diphenhydramine that was not included in the FDA's nighttime sleep aid monograph. The manufacturer filed an abbreviated new drug application with the FDA and received approval for its use as a sedative.[21]

Drug category and indications for use
OTC sedatives relieve sleeplessness caused by difficulty in falling asleep.

Mode of action
Antihistamines classified as first generation or sedating antihistamines produce their effect by an action in the CNS.

Warnings and precautions
If doxylamine does not provide relief of sleeplessness within 2 weeks, a physician should be consulted because a more serious condition may be the problem. If an individual has asthma, glaucoma, emphysema, chronic pulmonary disease, shortness of breath, or difficulty in urinating because of an enlarged prostate, a physician should be consulted. Alcoholic beverages should not be drunk while taking doxylamine. If an individual is taking other sedatives or tranquilizers, a physician should be consulted before using this drug.[21]

Recommended dose
Adults and children over 12 years of age may take a single dose of 25 mg doxylamine 30 minutes before bedtime.

Product
Doxylamine (Unisom Sleep Tabs).

Combination sedatives and analgesics

Drug category and indications for use
The FDA has approved the combination of nighttime sedatives with oral analgesics to relieve occasional sleeplessness.

Mode of action
Mild discomfort and pain may prevent individuals from falling asleep easily, and the combination of an analgesic and sedative may be more beneficial than a sedative by itself.

Warnings and precautions
Acetaminophen, aspirin, or ibuprofen may be combined with diphenhydramine. Warnings and precautions for each active ingredient must appear on the label of the product.

Recommended dose
Adults and children over 12 years of age may take a single dose of 1000 mg acetaminophen with 50 mg diphenhydramine hydrochloride 30 minutes before bedtime. Adults and children over 12 years of age may take a single dose of 1000 mg aspirin with 72 mg diphenhydramine citrate 30 minutes

before bedtime. Adults and children over 12 years of age may take a single dose of 400 mg ibuprofen with 72 mg diphenhydramine citrate 30 minutes before bedtime.

Products
Acetaminophen and diphenhydramine (Tylenol PM), aspirin and diphenhydramine (Bayer Aspirin PM), ibuprofen and diphenhydramine (Advil PM).

Dietary supplements

Melatonin

Although melatonin is a human hormone, it is not regulated as an OTC drug by the FDA. It is available from animal sources or from a chemical synthetic process as a dietary supplement. The body synthesizes melatonin through several metabolic steps beginning with the conversion of the amino acid tryptophan to serotonin and ultimately to melatonin.

Numerous studies have been conducted to determine the efficacy of melatonin as a sleep aid. Although many clinical trials reported positive results compared with placebos, the results were not statistically significant in many studies.[22] Most of the clinical trials had small numbers of patients and were for short durations of use.

The evidence for the use of melatonin for jet lag in travelers has some positive results for travel in an eastward direction if travel was through three to five time zones, but the requirement for precise timing of dosing melatonin for at least 3 days before the scheduled trip may limit its usefulness.[22–24] Melatonin when combined with light therapy is more effective in altering an internal circadian rhythm mechanism, but self-care is not appropriate because it involves situations where insomnia is long term, not short term.[24]

Mode of action
Administration of exogenous melatonin elevates normal circulating levels of melatonin, especially in individuals who have levels less than normal blood concentrations, and it helps to relieve occasional insomnia. It acts at the same receptor sites in the brain as endogenous melatonin.[25]

Warnings and precautions
Melatonin has no serious adverse effects but may cause fatigue, headache, dizziness, and irritability, especially when higher doses are used (more than 3 mg).

Recommended dose
Adult doses for falling asleep should be 1 to 3 mg 30 to 60 minutes before bedtime. Adult doses for preventing jet lag are 1 to 3 mg taken at the projected time of the new sleep pattern, beginning 3 days before travel.

Products
Melatonin (Melatonex and many generic manufacturers).

Valerian

Valeriana officinalis is the source of extracts that contain valepotriates, sesqui-terpenes, and amino acids that are used in dietary supplements promoted as sleep aids. However, the type of preparation used (tablets of valerian extracts, teas or liquid preparation) vary greatly in the quantity of the compounds that are in the product. There are many fewer studies reported on the effectiveness of valerian, but the results, like those for melatonin, show slight benefit for insomnia when compared with placebos.

Mode of action
The exact mechanism by which valerian causes sedation is not known, but it may bind to gamma-aminobutyric acid (GABA) receptors, which normally reduce brain stimulation. It does not exert its full effect unless it is taken for 2 to 4 weeks. This certainly exceeds recommendations for occasional drowsi-ness, but it should be remembered that dietary supplements are not held to the rigorous standards of OTC drugs because they are not approved for use by the FDA.

Warnings and precautions
Reported adverse effects include GI upset, headache, and morning drowsiness.

Recommended dose
One cup of valerian tea made from a root extract is recommended several times a day. Tablets containing 500 to 1000 mg valerian root extract may be taken 1 hour before bedtime. An alcoholic liquid extract is available and the recommended dose is 15 to 20 drops.[26]

Product
Valerian (Alluna).

Stimulants

The only OTC drug used as a stimulant is caffeine, but many brewed coffees and teas, or energy drinks, may contain more caffeine than that permitted by the FDA in OTC drugs. Guarana is a plant source of caffeine that appears in many energy or natural products. Table 5.6 lists the amount of caffeine available in some popular beverages and energy drinks.

Drug category and indications for use
Stimulant drugs produce an effect in the CNS that helps to alleviate occasional drowsiness and fatigue and to increase mental alertness.[27]

Table 5.6 Caffeine content of popular beverages and energy drinks[a]		
Product	Usual size (ounces)	Caffeine content (mg)
Plain, brewed coffee	8–12	60–120
Plain, brewed, decaf coffee	8–12	< 10
Dunkin' Donuts	16	143
MacDonald's Large	16	145
Starbucks Coffee Grande	16	330
Starbucks Grande Cappuccino	16	150
Starbucks Grande Caffe Latte	16	150
Starbucks Espresso	1.5	77
Plain, brewed tea	8–12	20–90
Lipton Brisk Ice Tea	20	50
Snapple Iced Tea	16	42
Starbucks Tazo Chai Tea	12	75
Nestea Ice Tea	16	34
Coca-Cola	12	35
Diet Coke	12	45
Barq's Root Beer	12	23
Mountain Dew	12	55
Dr. Pepper	12	41
Pepsi	12	38
Full Throttle	16	144
TAB Energy	10.5	95
Jolt	23.5	280
Vault	12	70
So-Be Adrenaline Rush	16	152
So-Be No Fear	16	174
Rockstar	16	160
Red Bull	8.3	80
Propel Invigorating Water	20	50
Vitamin Water Energy	20	40

[a] Caffeine in drinks: http://www.energyfiend.com/the-caffeine-database (accessed: February 28, 2009).

Caffeine appears in many headache remedies because it increases the pain-relieving effect of OTC analgesics (see earlier discussion in this chapter). Caffeine also produces a mild diuretic effect and is used for this purpose in products that treat symptoms associated with premenstrual tension (Chapter 6).

Monograph drugs
Caffeine is the only approved monograph drug.

Mode of action
Caffeine stimulates the release of neurohormones, norepinephrine and epinephrine, in the brain, which increase mental alertness and ward off feeling of tiredness and fatigue.

Warning and precautions
Ingestion of caffeine from other sources should be limited when using a caffeine product to prevent nervousness, irritability, insomnia, and rapid heart beat. The product contains approximately as much caffeine as a cup of coffee. If drowsiness or fatigue persists, a physician should be consulted.[27]

Recommend dose
Adults and children over 12 years of age may take 100 to 200 mg of caffeine every 3 to 4 hours.

Products
Caffeine (NoDoz Maximum Strength, Ultra Pep-Back, Vivarin).

Antidepressant dietary supplements

St. John's wort

Diagnosis and treatment of depression is not a self-care problem and the FDA has not approved any OTC drugs for depression. However, individuals who think they are depressed may try taking OTC stimulants or dietary supplements such as St. John's wort. St. John's wort is widely used in Europe as an antidepressant, particularly in Germany. It is a dietary supplement in the USA and its sale does not require FDA approval. It is commonly used to treat mild to moderate depression.

Clinical trials comparing St. John's wort with placebo and low-dose tricyclic antidepressant drugs have demonstrated a positive effect, and it has fewer adverse effects than the tricyclic antidepressants.[28]

Drug category and indications for use
St. John's wort is a flowering plant or shrub whose extracts are used to promote a positive mood.

Mode of action
Products of St. John's wort are standardized based on the concentration of hypercin present in the product. Hypericin has weak effects by inhibiting the

reuptake of several neurotransmitters in the brain, including serotonin, norepinephrine and GABA. The plant also contains flavonoids, which contribute to its effect.[29,30] St. John's wort affects liver enzymes, especially cytochrome oxidase (CYP3A4).

Warnings and precautions
If individuals are taking other medications physician should be consulted because St. John's wort has many drug interactions. It decreases the effect of many drugs, including protease inhibitors and nonnucleoside reverse transcriptase inhibitors (used to treat HIV infections), oral contraceptives, cyclosporine, simvastatin, and warfarin. A sunscreen should be used when going outdoors because this product causes photosensitivity reactions.[29,30]

Because this drug is a dietary supplement, it must contain the following statement: 'This product has not been evaluated by the Food and Drug Administration. This product is not intended to diagnose, treat, cure, or prevent any disease.'

Recommended dose
The daily dose for adults is 300 mg three times a day. This product is not recommended for children. It may take up to 2 months for St. John's wort to produce its full effect.[30]

Case study exercises

Case 1 A 48-year-old woman tells the pharmacist that she uses two tablets of Tylenol Extra Strength (500 mg of acetaminophen per tablet) four times a day because she fell and her back is sore. She wants to know if she should use Tylenol PM to help her sleep better.
The pharmacist advises her not to use Tylenol PM because she is already taking the maximum recommended daily dose of acetaminophen. If she exceeds the recommended daily dose, she increases the risk of damaging her liver. If she is having trouble falling asleep, she could take a nighttime sedative containing diphenhydramine, such as Nytol, Sominex, or Simply Sleep.

Case 2 The mother of an 11-month-old infant asks the pharmacist what dose of Tylenol Infant Drops she should give the baby because the baby is teething and is cranking and crying.
The pharmacist tells the mother that Tylenol Infant Drops should not be administered to a child less than 2 years of age unless the doctor has advised her to do so. She could purchase a topical product such as Anbesol, which contains a local anesthetic, that is rubbed on the gums to relieve teething pain. (See Chapter 7.)

Case 3 A 56-year-old man who is not under the care of a doctor asks the pharmacist what dose of aspirin he should take to reduce the risk that he could have a heart attack. He is overweight like his father, who died from a heart attack.

The pharmacist recommends that he see a physician because using aspirin for a potential cardiovascular problem is not a decision that should be made by an individual. There are risks associated with the use of aspirin that must be evaluated before he should take aspirin on a daily schedule. The pharmacist explains that he should see a physician because he is overweight, and his father's health history may increase the risk he has for cardiovascular disease.

Case 4 A 44-year-old man had minor dental surgery done and the dentist recommended that he take an OTC anti-inflammatory drug such as ibuprofen for the moderate pain that he is having. He asks the pharmacist if there is some other drug that he could take that does not have to be taken every 4 hours because his job is such that he can't take the medication that frequently.

The pharmacist explains that naproxen sodium (Aleve) is the same type of drug as ibuprofen and has a longer duration of action and would solve his problem. It may be used twice a day.

Case 5 The mother of a 9-year-old girl tells the pharmacist that her daughter has a dance performance in a week and she is too excited and nervous to fall asleep. She asks if using valerian tablets (Alluna) would be suitable because it's a natural product.

The pharmacist advises her not to use any nighttime sedative because sedatives should not be used in children under 12 years of age without a doctor's recommendation. He also tells her that valerian would not be helpful because it takes approximately 2 weeks for it to have its optimum effect. He discusses methods to have the child get ready for bed at a set time and to have her avoid excitement and any beverages like cola drinks that contain caffeine in the late afternoon and evenings.

Case 6 A worker has just had a job change and complains of problems falling asleep at night. When he gets up in the morning, he feels tired and has no energy. He wants to know if Vivarin will help to give him energy during the day.

The pharmacist discusses the man's use of coffee and tea during the day. The man usually gets a 16 ounce Starbucks Grande Coffee on his way to work but he doesn't think it helps him with his fatigue. The pharmacist explains that Vivarin contains 200 mg caffeine and the

Starbucks coffee he drinks contains 330 mg caffeine. The pharmacist suggests that he not consume more caffeine since the coffee he drinks doesn't help him.

The pharmacist discusses an alternative of using a nighttime sedative such as diphenhydramine (Nytol, Sominex or Simply Sleep) or doxylamine (Unisom) for several nights. Perhaps he has some anxiety because of his new job and a few nights of a more restful sleep will help him. If this suggestion isn't satisfactory, he should see his doctor.

Case 7 The mother of a 15-year-old girl asks the pharmacist which OTC migraine drug would be best for her daughter.
The pharmacist discovers that the daughter has never seen a doctor about her headaches. The pharmacist tells the mother that OTC migraine products are only intended for use in individuals who are over 18 years of age and who have been diagnosed as having migraine headaches. The pharmacist recommends contacting the doctor and suggests using acetaminophen or ibuprofen as soon as the headache symptoms occur. The dosing directions on the product label should be followed until the appointment with the doctor.

References

1. Internal analgesic, antipyretic, and antirheumatic drug products for over-the-counter human use; tentative final monograph. *Fed Regist* 1988; 53: 46204–46260.
2. *Managing Migraines.* www.fda.gov/fdac/features/2006/206_migraines.html (accessed February 21, 2009).
3. Burke A *et al.* Analgesic-antipyretic and anti-inflammatory agents; pharmacotherapy of gout. In: Brunton LL *et al.* eds. *Goodman & Gilman's The Pharmacological Basis of Therapeutics*, 11th edn. New York: McGraw-Hill, 2006: 671–715.
4. *Health Bulletin: Use Caution With Pain Relievers.* Updates October 30, 2007. www.fda. gov/cder/consumerinfo/acetaminophen.htm (accessed February 5, 2009).
5. Internal analgesics, antipyretics and antirheumatic drug products for over-the-counter human use; proposed amendment of the tentative final monograph; required warnings and other labeling. *Fed Regist* 2006; 71: 77314–77352.
6. Organ-specific warnings; internal analgesic, antipyretic, and antirheumatic drug products for over-the-counter human use: final monograph. *Fed Regist* 2009; 74: 19385–19409.
7. FDA Panel Backs 'Black Box' Warnings for Acetaminophen Prescription Combos. http:// www.medpagetoday.com/ProductAlert/OTC/14922 (accessed July 12, 2009).
8. Schulman S. Hemorrhagic complications of anticoagulant and thrombolytic treatment: American College of Chest Physicians Evidence-Based Clinical Practice Guidelines (8th edition). *Chest* 2008; 133(Suppl 6): 257S–298S.
9. Labeling for oral and rectal over-the-counter drug products containing aspirin and non-aspirin salicylates; Reye's syndrome warning. *Fed Regist* 2003; 74: 18861–18869.
10. NINDA. *Reye's Syndrome Information Page.* www.ninds.nih.gov/disorders/reyes_ syndrome/reyes_syndrome.htm (accessed May 26, 2009).
11. Bennett WM, DeBroe ME. Analgesic nephropathy: a preventable renal disease. *N Engl J Med* 1989; 320: 1269–1271.
12. Naughton CA. Drug-induced nephrotoxicity. *Am Fam Physician* 2008; 78: 743–750.

13. New Information for Healthcare Professionals; Concomitant Use of Ibuprofen and Aspirin. www.fda/gov/cder/drug/Infosheets/HCP/ibuprofen_aspirinHCP.htm (accessed February 5, 2009).

14. *Advil Migraine Product Information.* www.Advil.com.products/migraine/migraine_label.asp (accessed February 21, 2009).

15. Internal analgesic, antipyretic, and antirheumatic drug products for over-the-counter human use; proposed amendment of the tentative final monograph, and related labeling. *Fed Regist* 2002; 67: 54139–54159.

16. *Aleve Labeling.* www.aleve.com (accessed February 21, 2009).

17. *Excedrin Migraine Product Information.* www.excedrin.com/prodGuide-migraine-label.shtml (accessed February 21, 2009).

18. Tibbitts GM. Sleep disorders: causes, effects, and solutions. *Prim Care Clin Office Pract* 2008; 35: 817–837.

19. Nighttime sleep-aid drug products for over-the-counter human use; final monograph; final rule. *Fed Regist* 1989; 54: 6814–6827.

20. Labeling of diphenhydramine containing drug products for over-the-counter human use. *Fed Regist* 2002; 67: 72555–72559.

21. *Unisom Drug Facts.* www.Unisom.com/DrugFacts.asp?product=10 (accessed February 24, 2009).

22. Buscemi N *et al. Melatonin for Treatment of Sleep Disorders. Summary, Evidence Report/Technology Assessment*: Number 108. [AHRQ Publication number 05-E002-1.] Rockville, MD: Agency for Healthcare Research and Quality, 2004 http://ahrq.gov/clinic/epcsums/melatsum.htm (accessed February 20, 2009).

23. Srinivasan V *et al.* Jet lag: therapeutic use of melatonin and possible application of melatonin analogs. *Travel Med Infect Dis* 2008; 6: 17–28.

24. Sack RL *et al.* Circadian rhythm sleep disorders: Part I. Basic principles, shift work and jet lag disorders. *Sleep* 2007; 30: 1460–1483.

25. Gooneratne NS. Complementary and alternative medicine for sleep disturbances in older adults. *Clin Geriatr Med* 2008; 24: 121–138.

26. Jellin JM *et al.* Valarian. In: *Pharmacist's Letter/Prescriber's Letter Natural Medicines Comprehensive Database,* 3rd edn. Stockton, CA: Therapeutic Research Faculty; 1999: 926–928, 1052–1054.

27. Stimulant drug products for over-the-counter human use; final monograph; final rule. *Fed Regist* 1988; 53: 6100–6105.

28. Linde K *et al.* St. John's wort for major depression. *Cochrane Database Syst Rev* 2008; (1): CD000448.

29. Wurglics M, Schubert-Zsilavecz M. *Hypericum perfortum*: a 'modern' herbal antidepressant. *Clin Pharmacokinet* 2006; 45: 449–468.

30. Schneider C, Korsen N. Complementary and alternative medical approaches to treating depression in a family practice setting. *Clin Family Pract* 2002; 4: 873–893.

6

Genitourinary system

This chapter discusses products affecting the urinary tract and gender-based products. There are very few urinary-tract conditions that are amenable to self-care because most require diagnosis by a physician, and appropriate therapy requires prescription drugs. The most common symptom that affects both men and women as they age is increased urinary frequency and the discomfort that may accompany urination.

Men generally begin to experience symptoms of urinary frequency after the age of 50 or 60 because of enlargement of the prostate gland. The urethra passes through the prostate gland and as the prostate tissue increases in size it causes obstruction of urine flow, causing incomplete emptying of the urinary bladder. This leads to the need to empty the bladder frequently. There are many other serious medical conditions, such as cancer, that cause similar symptoms, and an appropriate diagnosis and treatment requires physician supervision. However, many men are reluctant to see a physician and prefer to try the dietary supplement saw palmetto to alleviate their symptoms.

Women are more likely to experience urinary-tract infections than men because of the anatomic differences between the sexes. The urethra is much shorter in women and the risk of bacteria entering the urinary tract is increased. Many women have frequent reoccurrence of infections, and increasing fluid intake and the use of dietary supplements or beverages containing cranberries may provide symptomatic relief and prevent infection.

There are two drugs available for treatment of discomfort during urination for which the FDA has not issued a final ruling. Phenazopyridine is classified as a urinary analgesic drug, and methenamine is a urinary antiseptic (antibacterial). The FDA plans to issue a ruling that will clarify its position on the marketing of unapproved drugs that manufacturers will be required to follow.

Many women experience mild, temporary edema (fluid retention) along with other symptoms, including premenstrual tension and dysmenorrhea, during the menstrual cycle and the FDA has approved several OTC diuretics in a monograph for this purpose.

Contraception may be a concern to both sexes and condoms for men and women are available as OTC products. The use of condoms also reduces the risk of sexually transmitted diseases. Spermicidal products for vaginal use are also available as OTC products.

Many women are prone to develop a vaginal candida (yeast) infection, especially those who have diabetes or are taking broad-spectrum anti-biotics. The FDA permits the sale of OTC vaginal antifungal agents for women who have been previously diagnosed as having a candida infection by a physician.

Urinary-tract drugs

Urinary analgesics

Phenazopyridine

The FDA has not approved the efficacy claims of phenazopyridine as a urinary-tract analgesic but it has not taken any action to call for its removal from the marketplace at this time. The FDA has indicated that it intends to declare any OTC products as misbranded or adulterated if they do not have specifically approved drugs as active ingredients. These products will remain on the market until FDA takes a final action on this proposed policy, or until a manufacturer submits data proving efficacy. Phenazopyridine appears currently in several prescription drugs as a urinary analgesic in the USA.[1]

Drug category and indications of use
Phenazopyridine acts as a urinary analgesic to relieve the burning, discomfort, and pain that occurs during urination; it may relieve symptoms of urinary urgency and frequency.

Mode of action
The mechanism of action of phenazopyridine is not known, but it has no effect as a urinary antiseptic or antibacterial agent.[2]

Warnings and precautions
If an individual has kidney disease or glucose-6-phosphate dehydrogenase deficiency, this drug should not be used without consulting a physician. If a yellowing of the eyes or skin develops, or if fever, chills, confusion, back pain, blood in the urine occur, a physician should be consulted. Use of this drug should be limited to 2 days. If symptoms are not relieved or if they worsen, a physician should be called. Phenazopyridine will cause a red–orange color in the urine and may stain clothing. It will also stain soft contact lenses and these should not be worn while taking this drug.[2,3]

Recommended dose
Adults may take two tablets after each meal for 2 days with a full glass of water; not more than 12 tablets should be taken and the tablets should be swallowed not chewed.[3]

Products
Phenazopyridine (Azo-Standard, Uristat, UTI Relief, Uricalm).

Urinary-tract antiseptic (antibacterial)

Drug category and indications for use
Methenamine is bactericidal because of its antiseptic properties and helps to relieve urinary frequency and urgency associated with urinary-tract infections.[2]

Monograph ingredient
Methenamine.

Mode of action
In an acidic environment, menthenamine breaks down to form ammonia and formaldehyde, which kill microorganisms.

Warnings and precautions
A physician should be consulted the first time urinary pain, discomfort, and/or frequency are experienced. Adverse effects include upset stomach, vomiting, and diarrhea. The development of a skin rash or hives may indicate an allergic reaction to methenamine, and the physician should be called immediately.[4]

The product Cystex contains methenamine and sodium salicylate, which requires the following additional warnings.[5] 'If you are allergic to aspirin or any other analgesic drug do not take this product.' 'If you have peptic ulcer disease or bleeding problems do not take this product.' 'If you are on a salt restricted diet, do not take this drug.' 'If you are an adolescent who has recently had chickenpox or the flu, do not take this drug because it increases your risk of developing Reye's syndrome.'

Recommended dose
Adults and individuals over 12 years of age may take two tablets up to four times a day with food and a full glass of water. The tablets should not be chewed. If pain and discomfort persist for 10 days or worsens, a physician should be consulted.[5]

Products
Methenamine (Cystex, also contains sodium salicylate).

Dietary supplements

Cranberry

Indications for use
Cranberry juice or powered extracts may reduce the risk for urinary-tract infections for individuals who are likely to have recurrent infections.[6]

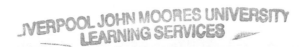

Mode of action

Cranberry products are not antibacterial agents but studies revealed that they reduce they ability of bacteria to adhere to the bladder wall. When fluid intake is increased, the population of bacteria in the bladder is reduced, preventing infections.

Warnings and precautions

High doses of cranberry may cause stomach irritation and diarrhea. Cranberries are very bitter and many natural cranberry drinks are sweetened with large quantities of sugar, which should be avoided by individuals who have diabetes and individuals who may be on weight-loss programs. Many beverages are now prepared with artificial sweeteners to avoid these problems.

There are reports that cranberry juice increases bleeding in patients taking warfarin, an anticoagulant. Individuals should consult their physician before consuming large quantities of cranberry juice if they are taking warfarin. Large quantities of cranberry products may increase the risk of kidney stones in individuals who previously had oxalate kidney stones.

Recommended dose

Adults and individuals over the age of 18 should drink 3 to 16 ounces (90–480 mL) of cranberry juice daily to prevent urinary-tract infections. If 300 or 400 mg of powered cranberry extract as tablets or capsules are used, the dose should be between one and six capsules twice a day with a large glass of water 1 hour before meals or 2 hours after meals.

Products

Ocean Spray Cranberry Juice and many others.

Urinary diuretics

Drug category and indications for use

Caffeine has mild diuretic activity and relieves mild edema (fluid retention) associated with the menstrual cycle. It may be labeled to reduce the temporary weight gain and breast tenderness associated with menstruation.[7]

Monograph ingredients

Caffeine and pamabrom (8-bromotheophylline) are chemically methylxanthine compounds. Ammonium chloride (NH_4Cl) is approved in the monograph but does not appear in current products.

Mode of action

Methylxanthines cause vasodilatation and a slight increase in renal blood flow and glomerular filtration rate. Sodium and chloride are excreted, increasing urine volume and reducing edema.[7]

Warnings and precautions
Caffeine's label must state that the product contains about the same caffeine content as a cup of coffee and intake of beverages with caffeine should be limited. Other caffeine-containing drugs should be limited because an overdose of caffeine is possible. Adverse effects include gastric irritation, rapid heart beat, increased blood pressure, irritability, nervousness, and insomnia.[7]

Pamabrom's label does not contain the same warnings because it does not have a stimulant effect like caffeine on the CNS and the cardiovascular system.[7]

Recommended dose
Caffeine may be used by adults and individuals over 12 years of age; 100 to 200 mg may be taken every 3 to 4 hours as long as symptoms persist.[7]

Pamabrom may be used by adults and individuals over 12 years of age as a 50 mg dose up to four times a day.

Products
Caffeine (used in many menstrual combination products); pamabrom (Aqua Ban and Diurex Aquagels).

Products for men

Dietary supplement diuretics

Drug category and indications for use
Certain compounds in juniper berries, buchu, uva ursi, sandalwood, couch grass, dandelion, and cubeb berries are claimed to have a diuretic action. These herbs also appear in many homeopathic products in concentrations much lower than those in dietary supplements.

Diurex For Men contains buchu, dandelion, juniper extract, and guarana, a natural ingredient containing caffeine, and is described as helping to support healthy fluid balance and aid in the elimination of excess body water and its related discomforts.[8]

Mode of action
Many plant compounds are excreted by the kidney and may act on the bladder to cause irritation, which may increase urination.

Product
Diurex Water Pills for Men.

Warnings and precautions
Diurex can be used by healthy men over 18 years of age. If any other medications are being taken, a healthcare professional should be consulted before using this product.[8]

As a dietary supplement, Diurex must contain the following statement on the label. 'These statements have not been evaluated by the FDA. This product is not intended to diagnose, treat, cure or prevent any disease.'

Dietary supplement for benign prostate hyperplasia

The first symptoms of benign prostatic hyperplasia (BPH) are a weaker urine stream, difficulty in initiating urine flow, and increased urinary frequency. The incidence of BPH increases with age. The appropriate recommendation for males who have these symptoms is an examination by a physician for a diagnosis, because these symptoms are also associated with prostatitis and cancer of the prostate.

BPH is most appropriately treated with prescription drugs. Relief of urinary frequency and urgency is achieved by using drugs that specifically inhibit alpha-adrenoceptors in the urinary tract so that the bladder can be more completely emptied and the urine stream is more forceful.

Another way to manage this medical condition is to use drugs that block the enzyme 5-alpha-reductase. This enzyme is in the pathway for production of dihydrotestosterone, an androgenic hormone responsible for the growth of the prostate gland. Finasteride and dutasteride are two prescription drugs that inhibit this enzyme. Saw palmetto (*Serenoa repens*) produces the same effect but its activity is much weaker than the prescription drugs. The enzyme-inhibiting drugs may take up to 6 months to relieve BPH symptoms, and the degree of their effectiveness is related to the actual size of the prostate gland, which can only be determined by a physician. Comparison of saw palmetto with finasteride in men with mild to moderate symptoms showed similar relief of symptoms but no improvement in any objective measure of urinary or prostate health. Saw palmetto did have fewer adverse effects than finasteride. Saw palmetto has produced a positive effect in many placebo trials.[9,10]

Indications of use
Saw palmetto may be useful in maintaining prostate and urinary health.

Herbal ingredient
Saw palmetto.

Mode of action
Saw palmetto contains plant sterols that are weak inhibitors of 5-alpha-reductase and reduce the formation of dihydrotestosterone.

Warnings and precautions
Saw palmetto should not be taken by pregnant women or women who plan to become pregnant because of its potential antiandrogenic effect on the fetus. Saw palmetto may cause gastric irritation, nausea, constipation, and diarrhea.

It should be used with caution if anticoagulants such as warfarin are being used because it may increase bleeding. Bleeding has also been reported if it is used with ginkgo biloba.[10]

Saw palmetto is not recommended by the American Urological Association for treatment of BPH. The product label must carry the standard dietary supplement warning, 'This product is not intended to diagnose, treat, cure or prevent any disease.'

Male condoms

Condoms have a long history of use in the prevention of unwanted pregnancy, but their importance as a device that prevents sexually transmitted disease is a more recent development. Condoms made from natural rubber latex or polyurethane are effective in preventing infections that may be spread by contact with the head of the penis, such as HIV (AIDS), syphilis, and gonorrhea. They are less effective in preventing infections that are spread by contact with infected skin, for example human papillomavirus (HPV) or herpes virus. Condoms made from natural lamb intestines are effective in preventing pregnancy but not in preventing any sexually transmitted disease (STD). Condoms may also be used to collect semen to determine sperm count during fertility evaluations.

Condoms are effective because they are a physical barrier to sperm, bacteria, and viruses; they are unrolled over an erect penis, creating a sheath-like cover. Condoms may be purchased with or without a reservoir tip. When a condom without a reservoir tip is used, an area or space should remain at the tip of the condom to prevent rupture of the condom during ejaculation. Condoms are available with or without a lubricant, have varying thicknesses, and many designed surfaces and colors that are intended to enhance the sexual experience. Lubricants have not been evaluated or approved by the FDA.

If an individual or his partner is sensitive to latex, a polyurethane or lamb skin condom should be used. Some condoms use a spermicidal lubricant, but the amount of the lubricant is not deemed to be sufficient to kill all sperm. Lubricants that are used with condoms should not be oil or petroleum based (e.g. petrolatum (Vaseline)) because they may damage the condom.

Condoms should be stored in a cool, dry place. A condom that feels sticky or appears damaged should not be used. The FDA requires that each condom be tested to be certain that all standards are met during the manufacturing process.[11]

General directions for effective use of a condom include the following.[11] 'A condom should be used every time the individual has sex and may only be used once. Condoms must be stored properly and should not be used after its expiration date. Proper use of a condom requires that it be held at its base when withdrawing the penis to prevent spillage of the ejaculate; dispose of the

Table 6.1 Pregnancy rate (percentage in one year) using no contraception and common contraceptive methods

Contraceptive method	Perfect use (%)	Typical use (%)
None	85	85
OTC male condom	2	15
OTC female condom	5	21
OTC sponge no prior births (prior births)	9 (20)	16 (32)
Rx estrogen/progesterone	0.3	8
Rx injection (Depo-Provera)	0.3	3
Rx transdermal (Evra Patch)	0.3	8
Diaphragm	6	16

OTC, over the counter; Rx, prescription.
Adapted from Trussell J. Contraceptive efficacy. In: Hatch RA et al. eds. Contraceptive Technology, 18th edn. New York: Ardent Media, 2004.

used condom properly. If the condom breaks or leaks, the woman should use emergency contraception to prevent pregnancy.'

Directions for use of latex and polyurethane condoms include: 'Condoms help to prevent pregnancy and reduce the risk of transmission of HIV infection, AIDS, and many other STDs.'

Directions for use of lamb's skin condoms include: 'Condoms help to prevent pregnancy, but do not reduce the risk of STDs, including HIV and AIDS.'

Condoms are not 100% perfect in preventing pregnancy even when used properly. Both partners should use contraceptives to be more certain that pregnancy does not occur. Women may use OTC spermicidal agents or prescription devices such as a diaphragm, intrauterine device, cervical cap, or oral, transdermal, or injectable contraceptive. If a male condom is being used, the female should not use a female condom. Table 6.1 has the overall pregnancy rates expected with the various contraceptive measures.[12]

Products for women

Female condoms

The female condom is shaped like a cylinder; it is 7 inches (17 cm) long and has one closed end and one open end. Both ends contain a soft, flexible ring. The closed end is pushed together and inserted vaginally before intercourse so that it covers the cervix and the ring on the open end remains outside the vagina. It provides protection against pregnancy and STDs.[13]

The FDA has only approved one manufacturer of female condoms. There are two types of female condoms available. The FC Female condom is made of polyurethane and the FC2 is made of nitrile. If a lubricant is used, it should be water soluble, the same as for male condoms.

Directions for use of the female condom includes the following.[13] 'Insert the condom before intercourse, being certain the closed end covers the cervix and be careful not to tear the condom with fingernails or jewelry. A new condom is required each time the individual has intercourse, and do not use the condom if the expiration date has passed. Squeeze the open end of the condom together and twist it before removal to prevent spilling its content; dispose of the condom properly. If the condom tears during intercourse or the contents spill, consider using emergency contraception to prevent pregnancy.'

Vaginal spermicides

Drug category and indications for use
Vaginal spermicides are intended to prevent pregnancy.

Mode of action
Spermicides are nonionic surface-acting agents that disrupt the lipid membranes of sperm. They may be used alone or with diaphragms and condoms.[14]

Monograph drug
Nonoxynol 9 is the only monograph spermicide.

Warnings and precautions
Spermicides are intended for vaginal use only. The product does not protect against infections by HIV or other STDs. Nonoxynol 9 may cause irritation of vaginal tissue, which may increase the risk of getting HIV from an infected partner. If the individual or her partner has HIV/AIDS, another form of birth control is recommended (male latex or polyurethane condoms). The product may cause vaginal irritation, burning, or itching. If a rash develops in the individual or her partner, use of the product should be stopped and a physician should be consulted. A douche product should not be used for at least 6 hours after intercourse.[14]

Recommended dose

> *Directions for vaginal inserts.* 'The woman should use one vaginal insert 10 minutes before sexual intercourse; each insert provides one hour of protection.'
> *Directions for cream, jelly, or foam.* 'Insert the contents of one applicator into the vagina 10 minutes before intercourse; each dose provides one hour of protection.'

Directions for vaginal films. 'Use your finger to insert one contraceptive film vaginally so that it covers the cervix before intercourse; one film will provide up to 3 hours of protection.'

The contraceptive sponge has been available in the USA for varying periods of time. Its unavailability has never been caused by problems of safety or efficacy, but rather with problems in the manufacturing process, lack of approval of an abbreviated new drug application, or financial decisions made by the manufacturer. The sponge is scheduled to appear in the US market in the summer of 2009. The sponge is inserted vaginally to cover the cervix and may be left in place for 24 hours.

Products
Nonoxynol 9 (Ortho Options Delfen Vaginal Contraceptive Foam, Ortho Options Conceptrol Prefilled Vaginal Contraceptive Applicators, Encare Vaginal Contraceptive Inserts, VCF Vaginal Contraceptive Film, Today Sponge).

Emergency contraception

Levonorgestrel (Plan B)

The FDA originally approved OTC status for the sale of a package containing two tablets, each containing 0.75 mg levonorgestrel, as emergency contraception if purchased by someone 18 years of age or older.[15] The federal courts in the USA ordered the FDA to make Plan B available to those aged 17 years of age in spring 2009 because women of that age were included in the clinical trials. The FDA indicated that it intends to comply with the order.[16]

Drug category and indications for use
Progestin only tablets reduce the chance of pregnancy when a woman has unprotected intercourse or if there is failure of some form of contraception.

Rx–OTC switched drug: levonorgestrel
The FDA approved the switch of levonorgestrel, a progestin, to OTC status, but it may only be purchased from a pharmacist as a behind-the-counter drug.

Mode of action
Progestin therapy may prevent release of the ovum if taken before ovulation or it may prevent fertilization from occurring. It may also prevent implantation of a fertilized ovum in the uterus.[15]

Warnings and precautions
Women who are pregnant should not use levonorgestrel because it is not effective if they are already pregnant. It should not be used as a routine form of contraception. The woman's next menstrual cycle should occur within 3 days of the expected date. If menstruation is more than a week late, the woman should consider taking a pregnancy test.

Levonorgestrel does not provide any protection from STDs. Adverse effects include nausea, vomiting, abdominal discomfort or pain, fatigue, headache, alteration in the amount of bleeding during the period, and breast tenderness.[16]

Recommended dose
Levonorgestrel is most effective when taken within 72 hours after unprotected intercourse. One tablet of levonorgestrel 0.75 mg should be taken as soon as possible and the second tablet should be taken 12 hours later. The greater the time elapsed between intercourse and taking the first dose, the less effective the drug is in preventing pregnancy.

If vomiting occurs within 1 to 2 hours after taking the first tablet, the dose must be repeated and a second dose must be taken 12 hours later. (Since the package contains only two tablets, if the woman vomits after the first tablet, a second purchase may be necessary because two doses of levonorgestrel are necessary for the drug to be effective.) The cost of Plan B (two tablets) is around $40.00.

Product
Levonorgestrel (Plan B: Next Choice (available in Fall 2009; newly approved generic)). NOTE. On July 16, 2009 the FDA approved Plan B One Stage which contain 1.5 mg of levonorgestrel in one tablet instead of the two tablet dose.

Vaginal antifungal drugs

Vaginal infections are not unusual in women once menarche occurs. Overgrowth of *Candida albicans*, a normal inhabitant of the vagina, is the most frequent cause of vaginal infections. Women who have diabetes mellitus are at greater risk for infection, as are women who are immunosuppressed or who take broad-spectrum antibiotics or oral contraceptives. Sanitary pads should be changed frequently during menstruation and tampons should not be used.[17]

Cleansing the vaginal area and keeping it dry are helpful in preventing candida infections. Many women cleanse the vagina by using douche products. There are no specific medical recommendations for using douches in normal healthy women. These products are not evaluated by the FDA; they contain surfactants for cleansing and may have buffers and pH adjuster to help to maintain the normal environment in the vagina.

There is some evidence that ingestion of probiotic nutrients in yogurts, those having live lactobacilli or bifidobacteria, may help to prevent vaginal yeast infections. The FDA has not approved the use of the probiotics for this purpose.

The symptoms associated with yeast infections include vaginal itching and a thick, white, discharge that looks like cottage cheese. Once a woman has had a candida infection that was diagnosed by a physician, she may choose to treat her next candida infection with an OTC vaginal antifungal drug.

Drug category and indications for use
Candida or yeast infections are treated with topical, vaginal antifungal drugs. Vaginal antifungal drugs relieve itching and irritation caused by the vaginal yeast infections.

Rx–OTC switched drugs
Butoconazole, clotrimazole, miconazole, and tioconazole are all approved for use as vaginal antifungal drugs.

Mode of action
All of the OTC antifungal drugs are classified chemically as imidazoles. They bind to sterols in the fungal membrane, causing changes in its permeability that result in fungal cell death.[18]

Warnings and precautions
These products should not be used if a woman is pregnant. A woman should not use this product if she has never had a vaginal yeast (candida) infection diagnosed by a physician. The product should not be used if lower abdominal, back or shoulder pain is present; if fever or chills, nausea, or vomiting develop; or if a foul-smelling vaginal discharge is present.[17]

A woman should not have vaginal intercourse when using a vaginal anti-fungal drug. This product may damage condoms and diaphragms and should not be used with tampons, douches, spermicides, or other vaginal products. These drugs provide no protection against STDs.

If there is no relief of symptoms within 3 days of using this product, or if the symptoms last longer than 7 days, the woman should consult a physician.[17]

Recommended dose
Adults and children over 12 years of age may use vaginal antifungal drugs. Products are available that are to be used for 1, 3, or 7 days. The concentration of the active drug differs for each type of product, with the single-day treatments having the highest concentrations and the 7-day treatments having the lowest concentration. Vaginal products may be suppositories (inserts) or vaginal creams that are to be used once daily before bedtime. Formulations consisting of a vaginal cream come with an applicator that is inserted vaginally, depressing a plunger delivers the cream to the vagina. Some products come in prefilled, disposable applicators.

Products are also available as a topical cream for application to the skin around the vagina that may be irritated and itchy, and they may be used twice a day. Topical creams are to be used in addition to the formulation that is inserted vaginally.

Products

Clotrimazole (Gyne-Lotrimin 3 Vaginal Cream and Gyne-Lotrimin 7 Vaginal Cream), tioconazole (Monistat 1 Day Treatment and Vagistat-1), and miconazole (Monistat 1 Day Treatment Day or Night Combination Pack, Monistat 3 as vaginal suppositories (ovule inserts) or combination pack with inserts and topical cream, Monistat 7 Day Treatment with disposable applicators or as a combination with applicators and topical cream, Vagistat 3 as vaginal suppositories (inserts)).

Premenstrual and menstrual symptoms

Premenstrual syndrome comprises multiple symptoms, including bloating or edema, cramps, headache, backache, fatigue, and feelings of irritability, depression, and anxiety.

OTC drugs

The symptoms of cramps (lower abdominal pain) and headache may be treated using OTC analgesics, as discussed in Chapter 5. Bloating and edema may be treated using OTC diuretics, as discussed earlier in this chapter. Irritability, depression, and anxiety may be treated by using pyrilamine, an antihistamine. Since this is not a final monograph, pyrilamine, is permitted in products because the FDA has not made a final decision on its efficacy, but, it may only be used in a combination product to treat premenstrual or menstrual symptoms.

All of the above drugs have already been discussed, and table 6.2 contains a list of combination products available for premenstrual or menstrual symptoms.

Table 6.2 Content of combination products for relief of premenstrual or menstrual symptoms[a]

Product name	Analgesic	Diuretic	Pyrilamine
Diurex Advanced Water Pills	Magnesium salicylate	Caffeine	None
Diurex PMS Formula	Acetaminophen	Pamabrom	Yes
Pamprin Cramp	Acetaminophen and magnesium salicylate	Pamabrom	None
Pamprin Max	Acetaminophen and aspirin	Caffeine	None
Pamprin Max Multisymptom	Acetaminophen	Pamabrom	Yes
Premsyn pms	Acetaminophen	Pamabrom	Yes
Midol Max Strength Menstrual Complete	Acetaminophen	Caffeine	Yes
Tylenol Women's Menstrual Relief	Acetaminophen	Pamabrom	No

[a] Information obtained from product labels.

Menopausal symptoms

Perimenopause and menopause are associated with a series of symptoms that includes hot flushes (hot flashes), irritability, and difficulty in concentrating and sleeping. These symptoms are associated with the decrease in estrogen and progesterone as women reach their 40s and 50s. Many women use prescription hormone replacement therapy, but doing so slightly increases the risk of breast cancer. Many women seek alternatives, and herbal products are among these choices.

Dietary supplements

The National Center for Complementary and Alternative Medicine and the National Institute on Aging sponsored a study to evaluate the effect of black cohosh (*Actaea racemosa* and *Cimicifuga racemosa*) on the vasomotor symptoms associated with menopause, hot flashes, and night sweats. Black cohosh was used alone or combined with other herbal ingredients and compared with conjugated equine estrogens (with and without progesterone) and placebo. There was no difference between black cohosh alone or with other herbal ingredients and the placebo in relieving menopausal symptoms. The conjugated equine estrogen drugs did have a positive effect.[19,20]

Drug category and indications

Phytoestrogens (plant estrogens) are used to support the healthy, natural changes that occur during menopause.

Herbal ingredients

Black cohosh, soy and red clover are promoted for menopause health.

Mode of action

Phytoestrogens are purported to act at estrogen receptors in the body and to replace natural estrogen, which is declining. Phytoestrogens have a weaker action than human estrogens and are assumed to be safer than prescription drug hormone replacement therapy. A more recent placebo-controlled study reported that black cohosh, botanical products and dietary soy had no effect on vaginal epithelium, endometrium, or reproductive hormones when compared with hormonal replacement.[21] This finding adds doubt as to whether or not phytoestrogens act as true estrogenic substances in humans.

Warnings and precautions

Black cohosh may cause gastric irritation and headache. Soy and red clover contain phytoestrogens, which may act at human estrogen receptors; therefore, women at increased risk of diseases associated with estrogen administration (e.g. breast, uterine, or ovarian cancer; endometriosis; or uterine fibroids) should not use these products without consulting their physicians.

Recommended dose

There are no true recommended doses for these products, but they should not be used in children. Doses are based on those used in studies or products that are commercially available. A usual dose of black cohosh is 20 mg of root extract, which contains 1 to 2 mg triterpenes, once or twice a day.

Soy and red clover contain isoflavones and concentrations vary from 50 mg to approximately 120 mg. Soy is available in many foods, including soy milk, tofu, and soy noodles. Daily soy intake may vary from 25 to 50 g.[22]

Products

Black cohosh (Remifemin and generic products are available from many generic companies), phytoestrogens (Promensil and Estroven).

Case study exercises

Case 1 Allison is 17 years old and asks the pharmacist to recommend a product because she experiences swelling of her hands and feet and some breast tenderness during her menstrual cycle.
The pharmacist asks about her use of caffeine products and learns that she usually drinks a cup of coffee in the morning, but has no other caffeine. The pharmacist explains that products containing caffeine and pamabron would be helpful. The pharmacist explains that both act in the same manner so she should use only one product during her next menstrual cycle to determine if she has any relief. The pharmacist recommends Aqua Ban or Diurex Aquagels; both products contain pamabron.

Case 2 Charles, a 67-year-old man, asks the pharmacist to recommend a product because he is experiencing urinary frequency and has to get up two or three times a night to urinate and this is disturbing his sleep.
The pharmacist discusses Charles' problem and recommends that he consult a doctor. Charles has had these symptoms for about 8 months, but until a couple of weeks ago he only got up once during the night to urinate. The pharmacist tells Charles that since his problem increased in severity, there are no OTC products that will provide immediate relief. The dietary supplement that many men use, saw palmetto, may provide some symptomatic relief but it takes a few months before it really has an effect. Only prescription medications can provide Charles with a more timely relief. Charles is also at an age when he should have a prostate examination by a doctor to be certain that he doesn't have a more serious problem than the expected enlargement of the prostate that occurs with age.

Case 3 A 15-year-old girl asks the pharmacist whether she should use Tylenol Tablets or Motrin IB for the cramps and back pain that she gets when she has her menstrual period.

The pharmacist recommends Motrin IB because it has been shown to be more effective for menstrual-related pain. Motrin IB contains ibuprofen, a nonsteroidal anti-inflammatory drug, which has a greater effect on inhibiting the peripheral prostaglandin synthesis that is responsible for most of the symptoms she is experiencing. Although Tylenol also affects prostaglandin synthesis, it has very little anti-inflammatory effect.

Case 4 Scott asks the pharmacist what he should do about skin irritation he experiences on his penis and genital area after he uses a condom.

The pharmacist discusses the issue with Scott and learns that he is using a latex condom. The pharmacist suggests that he might be sensitive to the latex and that he should use a polyurethane condom. If Scott still has a skin irritation problem he should consult a physician.

Case 5 Gina tells the pharmacist she wants to purchase Plan B but she can't find it on any of the shelves in the pharmacy.

The pharmacist informs Gina that Plan B is only available from the pharmacist and cannot be put on the store's shelves with other products.

Case 6 Miriam asks the pharmacist to recommend a product because she has vaginal itching and a thin vaginal discharge that has a bad smell.

The pharmacist asks Miriam if she ever had this problem before and if she saw a doctor. Miriam replies that she has not. Miriam needs a proper diagnosis for her problem. The pharmacist recommends that Miriam should consult a physician because the only OTC drugs available for vaginal infections are for a yeast (candida) infection that was previously diagnosed by a physician. The pharmacist also explains that the symptoms she describes are not those usually associated with a yeast infection.

Case 7 Rachael is a 47-year-old woman who asks the pharmacist to recommend a sleeping product because she gets up several times during the night because of sweating, which disturbs her sleep. She also experiences similar symptoms during the day but they are less bothersome.

The pharmacist discusses the fact that she is probably having these symptoms because of normal decreases in her hormone levels that occur during menopause. An OTC sedative may or may not help her sleeping problem, but it certainly would have no effect of the cause of her night sweats. The pharmacist suggests that she discuss the problem with her physician because she may want to consider hormone replacement therapy.

Rachael asks about herbal therapy because she is aware that hormone therapy could increase her cancer risks. The pharmacist suggests that she could increase soy in her diet or purchase dietary supplements of soy or red clover, which contain phystoestrogens, plant estrogens. Black cohash is another product that has been used for normal menopausal symptoms. He also tells Rachael that controlled clinical trials have not shown that these dietary supplements produce significant relief of night sweats, but they may provide some relief that could help her problem. If Rachael does not obtain relief, she should discuss the issue with her physician.

References

1. *Phenazopyridine*. www.nlm.nih.gov/medlineplus/druginfo/meds/a682231.html. Last reviewed September 1, 2008 (accessed March 3, 2009).
2. Petri WA. Sulfonamides, trimethoprim–sulfamethoxazole, quinolones, and agents for urinary tract infections. In: Brunton LL *et al.* eds. *Goodman & Gilman's The Pharmacological Basis of Therapeutics*, 11th edn. New York: McGraw-Hill, 2006: 1111–1126.
3. *Uricalm Label Information*. www.drugstore.com:80/products/prod.asp?pid=152874&catid=11647 (accessed March 3, 2009).
4. *Methenamine Information*. www.nlm.nih.gov/medlineplus/druginfo/meds/a682296.html (accessed March 3, 2009).
5. *Cystex Label*. http://drugstore.com.products/prod.asp?pid=159288catid=11647 (accessed March 7, 2009).
6. *Cranberry (*Vaccinium macrocarpon*) Information*. www.nlm.nih.gov/medlineplus/druginfo/natural/patient-cranberry.html (accessed March 5, 2009).
7. Orally administered menstrual drug products for over-the-counter human use; tentative final monograph; notice of proposed rulemaking. *Fed Regist* 1988; 46194–46202.
8. Diurex Pills for Men. www.Diurex.com (accessed March 5, 2009).
9. Edwards JL. Diagnosis and management of benign prostatic hyperplasia. *Am Fam Physician* 2008; 77: 1403–1410.
10. *Saw palmetto. (*Serenoa repens *[Bartram] Small) Information*. www.nlm.nih.gov/medlineplus/druginfo/natural/patient-sawpalmetto.html (accessed March 5, 2009).
11. *Labeling Guidance for Latex Condoms*. www.fda.gov/cdrh/comp/guidance/1688.html (accessed March 9, 2009).
12. Trussell J. Contraceptive efficacy. In: Hatch RA *et al. Contraceptive Technology*, 18th edn. New York: Ardent Media, 2004: 221–252.
13. *FC & FC2 Female Condom Label Information*. www.femalehealth.com/theproduct.html (accessed March 9, 2009).
14. Over-the-counter vaginal contraceptive and spermicide drug products containing nonoxynol 9; required labeling. *Fed Regist* 2007; 72: 71769–71785.

15. Vaginal contraceptive drug products for over-the-counter human use; establishment of a monograph; proposed rulemaking. *Fed Regist* 1980; 82014–82049.
16. *Plan B information.* www.fda.gov/cder/drug/infopage/planB/default.htm (accessed March 9, 2009).
17. *Guidance for Industry. Labeling Guidance for OTC Topical Drug Products for the Treatment of Vaginal Yeast Infections (Vulvovaginal Candidiasis).* www.fda.gov/cder/guidance/2483dft.pdf (accessed March 9, 2009).
18. Bennett, JE. Antifungal agents. In: Brunton LL *et al.* eds. *Goodman & Gilman's The Pharmacological Basis of Therapeutics,* 11th edn. New York: McGraw-Hill, 2006: 1225–1241.
19. *Menopausal Symptoms and CAM.* www.nccam.nih.gov/health/menopause/menopausesym[toms.htm (accessed February 19, 2009).
20. Newton KM *et al.* Treatment of vasomotor symptoms on menopause with black cohosh, multibotanicals, soy, hormonal therapy or placebo: a randomized trial. *Ann Intern Med* 2006; 145: 869–879.
21. Reed S *et al.* Vaginal, endometrial, and reproductive hormone findings: randomized, placebo-controlled trial of black cohash, multibotanical herbs, and dietary soy for vasomotor symptoms: the Herbal Alternatives for Menopause (HALT) Study. *Menopause* 2008; 15: 51–58.
22. *Product Review: Supplements for Menopausal Symptoms (Soy and Red Clover Isoflavones, Black Cohash, and Progesterone Cream).* www.ConsumerLab.com (accessed March 3, 2009).

7

Topical ophthalmic, otic, and oral cavity conditions

Topical ophthalmic products

There are several different OTC pharmacological products available to relieve common ophthalmic conditions, including dry eyes (artificial tears), irritated red eyes (astringents, vasoconstrictors, and antihistamines), cleansing (eye washes), and contact lens products. All ophthalmic products are sterile and buffered so that the osmotic pressure between ophthalmic fluids and the product are equal.

Single-use ophthalmic containers should be discarded after use. The tip of a multiuse container should not touch the eye, eyelid, or any other surface and should be capped immediately after use. Multiuse products contain preservatives that may cause irritation or allergic reactions in some individuals. Single-use containers should be used in these situations.

Certain symptoms are not amenable to self-care and require referral to a physician. These symptoms include eye pain, blurred or distorted vision, sensitivity to light, presence of foreign objects that cannot be removed by using eye washes, a copious thick discharge, and irritation and redness that worsen or persist for more than 72 hours.[1]

Conjunctivitis is a general term describing inflammation of the conjunctiva, the mucous membrane that lines the inner surface of the eye. This may result from irritation or from a viral or bacterial infection. There are no OTC products for ophthalmic infections.[2]

Blepharitis is an inflammation of the eyelids, and the most common causes are inflammation of hair follicles, irritation or blockage of sebaceous glands, and localized infection with *Staphlococcus aureus*, commonly referred to as a stye. These conditions are usually self-limiting, but some of the discomfort they cause may be relieved by applying warm compresses to the affected eye for 5 to 10 minutes several times a day. An ophthalmic lubricant ointment may also be useful.

Age-related macular degeneration, a serious eye disease, may be treated with high doses of antioxidants, eye vitamins, but these are oral products, not ophthalmic products.

Dry eye products (artificial tears)

The eye is constantly exposed to environmental conditions, such as wind, heat, and low humidity, causing the eyes to lose moisture. Tears are secreted by the lacrimal glands and act as both lubricant and cleansing agent. Tears are composed of lipids (cholesterol esters, phospholipids, triglycerides, and fatty acids) secreted mainly by sebaceous glands on the eyelids, aqueous compounds (electrolytes, primarily sodium and chloride, and other salts that act as buffering agents), and mucus (glycoproteins and mucopolysaccharides). These compounds protect the eyes from abrupt changes in osmotic pressure and pH. Lipids and mucus add viscosity to tears, which helps to retard evaporation and soothe mildly irritated eyes. Infrequent blinking causes dryness, and mild irritation and is frequently associated with wearing contact lenses for excessive periods of time or staring at computer or video screens.

Aging may be accompanied by decreased activity of the lacrimal glands and an alteration of the various components of tears. Medications such as anticholinergic drugs, antihistamines, diuretics, and some antidepressants also cause a decrease in tears. People who wear contact lenses may be bothered by dry eyes. Smoking may cause dry eyes and irritation and redness. Treatment for dry eyes is the use of artificial tear products, which are either demulcents or emollients.

Artificial tear solutions (demulcents)

Drug category and indications for use
Demulcents are water-soluble drugs that are instilled as liquid drops in the eyes to relieve dryness and mild irritation.

Monograph demulcent drugs
Cellulose derivatives (carboxymethylcellulose, hydroxyethylcellulose, hydroxypropylcellulose, and methylcellulose), dextran 70 (a water-soluble polymer), gelatin, polyols (polyethylene glycol (PEG) 300, PEG 400, polysorbate 80, and propylene glycol), and polyvinyl alcohol.[1]

Mode of action
Artificial tear solutions replace normal tears and provide lubrication to the eye, relieving discomfort.

Warnings and precautions
Liquid demulcents should not be used if they contain particulate matter or if the solution is cloudy or changed in color. If the condition worsens or persists

for more than 72 hours, use of the demulcents should be stopped and a physician consulted.

Recommended dose
One or two drops should be instilled in the affected eye as needed. Hands should be washed before using eye drop preparations. The proper method of using eye drops involves tilting the head backward, pulling the lower lid forward and placing one drop in the pouch-like area of the lower lid. Slowly return the lower lid to its normal position and close the eye for 1 to 2 minutes. Dry with a clean tissue if necessary. Repeat if a second drop is needed.

Products
Akwa Tears, GenTeal, Hypotears, Refresh, Systane, Tears Naturale, and Visine Tears.

Artificial tear ointments (emollients)

Drug category and indications for use
Emollients are lipid ophthalmic ointments applied to the lower eyelid to relieve dry eyes and minor irritations.

Monograph ingredients
Lanolin, anhydrous lanolin, light mineral oil, mineral oil, paraffin, petrolatum, white ointment, white petrolatum, white wax, and yellow wax.[1]

Mode of action
Emollients replace the normal lipid secretions from the sebaceous glands of the eyelids.

Warnings and precautions
If the condition worsens or persists for more than 72 hours, use of the emollient should be stopped and a physician consulted.

Recommended dose
Apply a thin amount of ointment to the lower eyelid. Wash hands, pull the lower eyelid down and apply a small amount of ointment (approximately one-quarter of an inch (0.5 cm)) to the inside of the lower eyelid.

Products
GenTeal Eye Ointment, Refresh P.M., and Stye Eye Ointment.

Eyewash solutions

An eyewash solution is intended to cleanse the eye and remove loose foreign matter and/or to relieve minor eye irritations, such as stinging and burning associated with dust, air pollution, and chlorinated water.

Drug category and indications for use
Eyewash solutions contain no pharmacologically active ingredients.[1]

Monograph drugs
Eyewashes or eye lotion contain water, agents to restore osmotic pressure, pH adjusters, buffers, and preservatives.

Mode of action
Washing the eye with a solution contained in an eyecup or flushing the eye with a solution that from a nozzle removes debris, liquid or solid, that accidentally enters the eye and causes discomfort. Eyewash solutions may be used to cleanse the eye of excess mucous secretions.

Warnings and precautions
Immediate medical treatment should be sought for all open wounds in or near the eyes or if noxious chemicals accidentally enter the eye.

Recommended dose
Products that have nozzles should be used while the individual bends over a sink and flushes the affected eye by squeezing the bottle gently with continuous pressure. When eye washes are used with eye cups, a clean eye cup should be filled half-way with solution. The cup is pressed against the skin surrounding the eye to prevent leakage of the eye wash. The eyelids should be opened to bath the entire eye.

Products
Collyrium, B&L Advanced Eye Relief, OcuFresh.

Hypertonic eye drops

Drug category and indications for use
A hypertonic solution contains a concentration of sodium chloride between 2% and 5%; this is greater than the 0.9% that is isotonic to the eye. It is used to reduce corneal edema.

Monograph ingredient
Sodium chloride solutions of 2% to 5% are approved drugs.

Mode of action
Addition of hypertonic sodium chloride to the eye causes a higher osmotic pressure in the eye, and excessive fluid in the cornea is removed as the eye attempts to equalize the osmotic pressures.

Warnings and precautions
These products should not be used except with the advice and supervision of a physician. If eye pain or changes in vision occur, or if the condition worsens or persists, a physician should be consulted. Temporary stinging and burning may occur.

Recommended dose
One or two drops are instilled in the affected eye as recommended by the physician.

Product
Muro-128.

Ophthalmic astringents

Drug category and indications for use
An astringent is instilled in the eye to help clear excess mucus, reducing irritation and discomfort.

Monograph ingredient
Zinc sulfate (0.25%) is the only approved astringent.

Mode of action
Astringents combine with protein, causing it to precipitate so that it may be removed from fluids in the eye.

Warnings and precautions
The product should not be used if it is cloudy or has changed color. A physician should be consulted if eye pain or changes in vision occur, or if the condition worsens or persists.

Recommended dose
One or two drops are instilled into the affected eye up to four times a day.

Product
Zincfrin (astringent, zinc sulfate, plus a vasoconstrictor, phenylephrine).

Ophthlamic vasoconstrictors

Drug category and indications for use
Vasoconstrictors act to reduce redness of the eye resulting from minor irritation.[1,3]

Monograph ingredients
Ephedrine, naphazoline, oxymetazoline, phenylephrine, and tetrahydrozoline.[1,3]

Mode of action
Small blood vessels in the eye dilate and cause redness. Topical application of ophthalmic sympathomimetic drugs constricts these blood vessels, reducing or eliminating the redness.[1,3]

Warnings and precautions
These products should not be used if they are cloudy or have changed color. The solutions may cause the eyes to dilate and should not be used by those

with narrow-angle glaucoma unless advised by a physician. Excessive use of these products may increase redness of the eye.[3]

Recommended dose
One or two drops are instilled in the affected eye up to four times a day. The product should not be used in children under 6 years of age.

Products
Naphazoline (Clear Eyes and B&L Moisturizing Drops), oxymetazoline (Visine LR), phenylephrine (generic), and tetrahydrozoline (Visine, Visine Advanced Relief, and Murine Tears Plus).

Ophthalmic antihistamines

Drug category and indications for use
Antihistamine ophthalmic products are intended to relieve irritation, itchy eyes, watery secretions, and redness caused by an allergic response.

Rx–OTC switched drugs
Pheniramine and ketotifen have been approved for use as ophthalmic antihistamine drugs to alleviate the symptoms associated with allergic conjunctivitis. Pheniramine is only used when it is combined with the vasoconstrictor naphazoline.[3]

Mode of action
The release of inflammatory products, especially histamine, from the antigen–antibody immune reaction produces increased tearing, redness, and irritation. The antihistamine in the ophthalmic drops binds to the receptors where histamine normal binds. This blocks histamine from activating these receptors, preventing tearing, vasodilatation of small blood vessels, and redness.

Ketotifen is used alone and acts by blocking the receptor for histamine and by preventing histamine release from mast cells.

Warnings and precautions
The products should not be used if they are cloudy or have changed color. These products should not be used if eye pain or changes in vision occur, or if the condition worsens or persists for more than 72 hours.

> *Pheniramine products.*[3] 'Individuals who have narrow-angle glaucoma should not use vasoconstrictors because the pupils may dilate and become enlarged, worsening vision. This is a temporary condition. Do not use in children under 6 years of age.'
> *Ketotifen products.*[4] 'Do not use for redness associated with contact lens use. If you wear contact lenses, remove the lenses and wait for at least 10 minutes before reinserting lenses after using ketotifen. Do not use in children under 3 years of age.'

Directions for use

Pheniramine is used as one to two drops up to three or four times a day.

Ketotifen is used as one drop every 8 to 12 hours, but not more than twice a day.

Products

Pheniramine (Naphcon A, Opcon A, and Vasocon A), ketotifen (Zaditor).

Contact lens products

Contact lens and the solutions used for their disinfection are consider as devices and not drugs by the FDA. Contact lenses are made of polymers that correct vision and should be fitted by an eye physician. Lenses are classified as either soft or rigid gas permeable (RGP). The polymers used are different for each type of lens and the disinfecting solutions must be chemically compatible with the lenses. Several different manufacturers make contact lenses and products that are compatible with the lenses.

Improper cleaning and disinfection of contact lenses may lead to serious eye problems, including infections that may cause blindness. These conditions include acanthameoba keratitis, giant papillary conjunctivitis, and fusarium keratitis. General procedures to be followed to minimize the risk of infection include the following: (1) always wash hands before inserting or removing lenses; (2) do not use nonsterile water or saline solutions for cleaning or storage of the lenses; (3) use sterile disinfecting solutions for cleaning and storing lenses and do not reuse the solution; (4) do not use products if the expiration date has passed; (5) clean the lens case and allow it to air dry between uses; (5) clean lenses by gently rubbing the surfaces, rinse, and then store in lens case; (6) store the lenses in the appropriate solution for the recommended period of time needed for proper disinfection before using the lenses.[5]

Products

Soft contact lenses: ReNu Multipurpose Daily Disinfecting Solution, Opti-FreeRepleniSH Multipurpose Disinfecting Solution, CIBA Vision Clean Care H_2O_2 Cleaning and Disinfection Solution.

RGP contact lenses: Boston Multiaction Solution w/Daily Protein Remover, Boston Conditioning Advance Solution.

Otic products

The external ear is a blind canal that is lined with epithelial skin. Cerumen (ear wax) is produced as the secretions from the sebaceous and sweat glands combined with epithelial skin cells that are being shed and replaced. Cerumen has a light-yellowish color and becomes darker when it is exposed to air and is oxidized. Exposure to air also causes cerumen to lose moisture and become harder, causing discomfort and impaired hearing if it is not removed.

NOTE: There are no FDA approved drugs for topical use for earache (ear pain). Ear pain should be evaluated by a physician, but use of an oral analgesic such as acetaminophen, aspirin, or ibuprofen may relieve pain symptoms temporarily. There are homeopathic earache drops that contain chamomilla, sulfur, and mercury solubilis sold as Similasan products. As homeopathic products they do not have to prove safety or efficacy to the FDA (see Chapter 1.)

Ear wax removal aid

Drug category and indications for use
Ear wax softeners are intended to help in removing ear wax by softening and loosening excessive ear wax.[6]

Monograph ingredients
Carbamide peroxide (6.5%) and anhydrous glycerin drops are placed in the ear and remain there for a period of time to soften excessive ear wax in the external ear canal.

Mode of action
Ear wax softening agents absorb moisture, which lubricates hardened ear wax for easier removal from the external ear canal.

Warnings and precautions
These products should not be used unless directed by a physician if there is drainage or discharge from the ear, tinnitus, ringing or buzzing in the ear, dizziness, ear pain, a perforated ear drum, ear tubes, or ear surgery. Cotton swabs should not be used in the ear.[6]

Directions for use
The head is tilted and 5 to 10 drops of solution are added to the affected ear in adults and children over 12 years of age; ear wax softeners should not be used in children under 12 years of age unless directed by a physician. The solution is kept in the ear by inserting cotton in the ear. Drops may be used twice a day and for a maximum of 4 days. If the earwax is not removed, a physician should be consulted.[6]

The excess wax is removed by flushing the ear with water at room temperature or warm, using an ear syringe. Water that is too cold or too hot may cause nausea and vomiting and/or dizziness.

Products
Carbamide peroxide (Debrox, Murine Wax Removal System; this product contains an ear syringe with the drug product).

Prevention of swimmer's ear

Drug category and indications for use
Water that remains in the external ear canal may causes discomfort, a feeling of fullness in the ear, and may impair hearing. Drugs that dry water-clogged ears may be used to relieve these symptoms and may help to prevent infections in the external ear.[7]

Monograph ingredient
Isopropyl alcohol (95%) in anhydrous glycerin is approved for drying water-clogged ears.

Mode of action
If water remains trapped in the external ear canal from swimming or showering, it may create conditions causing discomfort in the ear and favor the growth of microorganisms that cause infections. Drugs that absorb the water or change the environment of the external ear reduce the risk of an infection.

Warnings and precautions
Isopropyl alcohol is flammable and should be kept away from flames and fire. It should not be used without consulting a physician if there is pain, drainage/discharge from the ear, or dizziness, or by anyone who has had ear surgery.[7]

Directions for use
The head is tilted and four to five drops are instilled in the affected ear. A plug of cotton may be used to keep the solution in the external ear canal.

Products
Isopropyl alcohol and anhydrous glycerin (Swim Ear and Auro Ear).

Oral cavity products

Tooth decay, gingivitis, periodontitis, aphthous ulcers, and fever blisters are the most common problems that affect the oral cavity and frequently these cause a great discomfort and pain. There are a variety of products that can relieve the discomfort associated with these conditions, but maintaining good oral hygiene is the best way to prevent their occurrence.

Anticaries drugs

Dental caries (tooth decay) may be prevented by daily brushing and flossing of the teeth. There are several other factors that are important in maintaining healthy teeth. There is a genetic component that provides greater resistance to tooth decay in some individuals, but the environment in the oral cavity is very important.

The presence of food debris, especially sugars, enhances the growth of bacteria that constitute the normal flora in the oral cavity. A sticky film, plaque, is formed in the mouth and adheres to the teeth. Bacteria in the plaque remain in close contact with the teeth, producing acidic waste products that can demineralize the calcium hydroxyapatite in the teeth's hard enamel surface.

The enamel protects the softer dentin, which contains the blood supply and nerve structure, beneath its surface from bacteria. Once the enamel loses its hardness through demineralization, bacteria invade the dentin, causing destruction and producing pain and tooth loss.

The salivary glands secrete saliva, which contains buffers to keep the pH slightly acidic, usually between 6.5 and 7.0 in healthy adults; enzymes necessary for initiating the digestion of certain foods; and electrolytes (minerals) to maintain the integrity of the teeth's enamel surface. Saliva helps to protect the teeth from decay by diluting and neutralizing acids produced by bacteria in the oral cavity.

Secretion of saliva is controlled primarily by activation of the parasympathetic (cholinergic) nervous system. If there is impairment in the production of saliva, the incidence of tooth decay increases. Anticholinergic drugs inhibit salivary secretion, causing dry mouth (xerostomia) as an adverse effect. There are many artificial saliva products that may alleviate this condition, but they are not considered to be drugs in the monograph system. Oasis Dry Mouth, Biotene Dry Mouth and OraMoist are popular saliva substitutes.

Drug category and indications for use

An anticaries drug helps to prevent dental caries, a disease of the calcified enamel of the tooth that results in demineralization and destruction of the dentin and its structures.[8]

Monograph ingredients

Sodium fluoride, stannous fluoride, and sodium monofluorophosphate applied topically to the teeth through the use of mouth rinses or dentifrices (toothpastes) act as anticaries drugs.[8]

Oral supplements containing fluorides are prescription drugs. Communities with a public water supply that serves over 25 000 people may add fluoride to the drinking water supplies. The optimum concentration of fluoride in drinking water ranges from 0.7 to 1.0 parts per million.

Mode of action

The ingestion or topical application of fluoride ion to the enamel of teeth results in the formation of fluoroapatite, a substance that increases the hardness of the enamel, making it more resistant to demineralization from the action of bacteria.

Warnings and precautions

These products should be kept out of the reach of children under 6 years of age. Anticaries toothpastes and oral fluoride rinse formulations should not be swallowed after use but should be spit out. When an oral fluoride rinse is used, food and drink should not be consumed for at least 30 minutes after rinsing.

Anticaries products have size limitations depending on the specific fluoride ingredient present. The purpose of this limit is to reduce the risk of toxicity from the fluoride component in case of accidental ingestion. Toothpastes are limited to 276 mg of total fluoride, and oral rinses to 120 mg.[8]

Stannous fluoride products may produce surface staining, which is not harmful and can be removed by a dentist.

Directions for use

Adults and children over 2 years of age should brush the teeth thoroughly with toothpaste after every meal or at least twice a day. Children under 6 years of age should be supervised until they are capable of using the products properly.

Adults and children over 6 years of age should use an oral fluoride rinse once a day after thoroughly brushing their teeth. They should swish 10 mL of fluoride rinse around the teeth for 1 minute and then spit it out. Fluoride rinses are used in children under 6 years of age only if recommended by the physician or dentist.

Products

All toothpastes that are labeled as anticaries products contain fluoride. Popular brands include Crest, Colgate, Aquafresh, Rembrandt, Tom's of Maine Natural Product Toothpaste, Ultra Brite.

The teeth should be flossed with regular dental floss or tape after brushing to remove debris from around the gums line and between the teeth. Dental floss and dental tape are not reviewed in the FDA's monograph system.

NOTE: Toothbrushes are available in many styles, sizes, and bristle designs. The American Dental Association recommends using a soft, multi-tufted, nylon bristle brush.[9] Electric toothbrushes with timers may help some individuals, especially children, to brush for the proper amount of time to thoroughly clean the teeth. Electric toothbrushes are recommended for individuals who have motor impairment and cannot use a hand brush properly.

Anticaries oral rinses

ACT, Listerine Tooth Defense, Listerine Smart Rinse, Phos-flur, and Tom's of Maine Natural Anticavity Rinse.

Antiplaque and antigingivitis mouth rinses

Brushing and flossing the teeth are the most effective ways to remove plaque and other debris from the teeth. If plaque is not removed from the teeth, it will become calcified and harden. This harden plaque (calculus or tartar) should be removed by a dental health professional. Accumulation of plaque and calculus cause the gums to become inflamed and bleed, especially when brushing the teeth. The gum around the tooth is loosened and recedes, allowing penetrate of bacteria under the gum where they can attack the periodontal ligaments that are responsible for holding the teeth in place (periodontitis).

Drug category and indications for use
Drugs applied to the oral cavity as mouth rinses or dentifrices to retard or prevent gingivitis and plaque are antigingivitis and antiplaque agents. These claims include removal of plaque, prevention of gum disease, and reduction in swelling and redness of gums, and bleeding gums.[10]

Monograph ingredients
Stannous fluoride toothpaste, cetylpyridinium chloride rinse (0.045 to 0.1%), triclosan, and a combination of volatile oils in a mouth rinse (eucalyptol, menthol, methyl salicylate, and thymol) may make antiplaque and antigingivitis claims.

Mode of action
Antigingivitis and antiplaque agents inhibit the growth of bacteria in the oral cavity.

Warnings and precautions
If gingivitis, bleeding, or redness lasts for more than 2 weeks, the product should be stopped and a dentist consulted. Pain, swollen gums, pus from the gums, loose teeth, and increasing space between the teeth are symptomatic of serious gum disease and require consultation with a dentist. These products should be kept out of reach of children under 6 years of age.[10]

Recommended dose
Stannous fluoride and triclosan toothpastes can be used by adults and children over 2 years of age for brushing the teeth after every meal or at least twice a day. Children under 6 years of age should be supervised until they are capable of using the product properly.

Adults and children over 12 years of age should swish 20 mL of cetylpyridinium chloride or 20 mL of combined volatile oils mouth rinse around the teeth twice a day for 30 seconds and then spit out. The rinse is not swallowed. Children between 6 and 12 years of age should follow the same directions but must be supervised. Children under 6 years of age should not use this product unless advised to do so by the dentist or physician.

Products
Cetylpyridinium (Cepacol, Crest Pro-Health), triclosan (Total), combined volatile oils (Listerine).

Tooth desensitizers

Drug category and indications for use
A tooth desensitizer is a gel or toothpaste applied to teeth that helps to relieve pain or build resistance to pain caused by cold, heat, sweets, acids, or contact.[11]

Monograph ingredient
Potassium nitrate (5%).

Mode of action
A tooth desensitizer acts on the dentin in the tooth to block pain and discomfort from stimuli that do not normally elicit a painful response in individuals with normal teeth.

Warnings and precautions
Sensitive teeth may be an indication of a more serious problem that should be treated by a dentist. If relief is not experienced within 4 weeks, or if the problem gets worse, a dentist or physician should be consulted.[11]

Directions for use
Adults and children over 12 years of age should use 1 inch (2.5 cm) of toothpaste on a soft bristle toothbrush and brush for 1 minute twice a day. Consult a dentist for use in children under 12 years of age.

Products
Potassium nitrate (Denquel, Sensodyne, Promise).

Fever blister or cold sore

Fever blisters or cold sores (herpes labialis) are an infection caused by the virus herpes simplex type 1 (HSV-1). Herpes labialis is characterized by the eruption of a lesion along the lips or nose where the epithelial cells meet the mucous membrane of the mouth or nose, causing irritation, swelling, and pain. Once an individual has contracted the virus, there is always the risk of additional episodes because the virus migrates and remains dormant in the nerve ganglia until a stressful situation arises.[12]

Stressful triggers include such factors as ultraviolet light exposure (sunlight), poor nutrition, fatigue, fever, extremes of hot or cold weather, and other infections. The most common trigger is the common cold, hence, the name 'cold sore.' The virus is easily transmitted by kissing or by using objects contaminated with virus, such as lip balms or lipsticks.

Frequently, the individual experiences a prodromal event, such as tingling or a feeling of burning, before the lesion appears. The lesion fills with fluid, gets larger, forms a blister that finally ruptures to create an ulcerous area on the lip that forms a crust.[12]

The FDA has not approved any prescription antiviral drugs for OTC use because it believes that their indiscriminate use may lead to resistance, creating the same type of problems seen with many antibiotic drugs. OTC treatment relies on the use of drugs classified as skin protectants and oral cavity anesthetics/external oral analgesics for symptomatic relief of irritation, discomfort, and pain. The FDA also approved 10% docosanol as an OTC drug through a new drug application (NDA)[13] but rejected the use of the amino acid lysine as an effective for the treatment of fever blisters.[14]

Oral protectant and external analgesic (anesthetic) combinations

Drug category and indications for use
Skin protectants are applied topically to fever blisters to relieve dryness and soften crusts to relieve discomfort.[15]

Monograph ingredients
Allantoin, calamine, petrolatum, zinc oxide, and cocoa butter are used together or combined with external analgesics for treatment of fever blisters.[15]

Mode of action
Oral skin protectants are pharmacologically inert and provide a continuous film over irritated or injured tissue.

Warnings and precautions
If symptoms persist for more than 7 days or worsen, a dentist or physician should be consulted.

Products
Skin protectants plus external analgesics for the treatment of fever blisters (Anbesol Cold Sore Therapy, Campho-Phenique Cold Sore Scab Relief). Table 7.1 lists the ingredients in these products.

Table 7.1 Fever blister/cold sore products containing skin protectants and/or oral anesthetics/analgesics

Product	Skin protectant	Anesthetic/external analgesics
Anbesol Cold Sore Therapy	Allantoin, petrolatum	Benzocaine, camphor
Carmex Cold Sore		Menthol, camphor, phenol
Campho-Phenique Cold Sore Treatment		Camphor, phenol
Campho-Phenique Cold Sore Scab Relief	Petrolatum	Pramoxime
Zilactin L Cold Sore Relief		Benzyl alcohol

Oral external analgesics

Drug category and indications for use
External analgesics are applied topically to fever blisters for temporary relief of pain and itching.[15]

Monograph ingredients
External analgesic drugs are predominately local anesthetics. Benzocaine, benzyl alcohol, camphor, dyclonine, lidocaine, menthol, phenol, phenolate sodium, pramoxine, and resorcinol all have local anesthetic activity.[15]

Mode of action
Topical external analgesics block nerve transmission from noxious stimulus of the peripheral system.

Warning and precautions
Products should not be used if there is an allergy to any ingredient.

Products
See table 7.1.

Docosanol

Drug category and indications for use
Docosanol is used to treat fever blisters and shortens healing time.[13]

Mode of action
Docosanol applied topically as soon as symptoms of a fever blister occur prevents the herpes virus from entering epithelial cells.[16]

New drug application drug
The FDA has approved 10% docosanol for shortening the time required for treatment of fever blisters.

Warnings and precautions
Docosanol is applied topically only to the affected area; it should not be used in or near the eyes and or inside of the mouth. If the fever blister gets worse or does not heal in 10 days, a physician should be consulted.[13]

Directions for use
Adults and children over 12 years of age should apply docosanol on the affected area as soon as the first symptom of a fever blister occurs. It should be applied five times a day until the fever blister is completely healed.

Product
Docosanol 10% (Abreva).

Canker sores or aphthous ulcers

Minor injury to the oral mucosa may cause irritation, inflammation, and ulceration of the mucosa, resulting in discomfort and pain, especially when acid, salty, or spicy foods or beverages are ingested. Most of these injuries are self-healing and do not require further treatment, but good oral hygiene is necessary to prevent a more serious condition, such as infection, from occurring. Oral wound cleansing agents are available for this purpose. If an individual has recurrent aphthous ulcer stomatitis, referral to a physician or dentist is appropriate.

External anesthetic/analgesic monograph drugs are also useful in relieving discomfort and pain associated with canker sores.

Drug category and indications for use

Oral wound cleansers temporarily clean minor wounds or inflamed gums caused by dentures, dental appliances, dental procedures, or accidental injury. They also may be used to remove phlegm, mucus, or other secretion associated with a sore mouth.[17]

Monograph ingredients

Carbamide peroxide in anhydrous glycerin, hydrogen peroxide, sodium bicarbonate, and sodium perborate are approved drugs.

Mode of action

Oral wound cleansers release oxygen when used as oral mouth rinses, loosening debris that is removed when the solutions are expectorated.

Warnings and precautions

If symptoms are not relieved in 7 days, or worsen, a dentist or physician should be consulted.

Directions for use

Adults and children over 2 years of age may use these products as a mouth rinse. The solution should be swirled around the mouth for 1 minute and then spat out for up to four times a day. Use of this product by children between 2 and 12 years of age requires supervision by a caregiver.[17]

Products

Carbamide peroxide (Gly-oxide, Cankaid), hydrogen peroxide (Peroxyl Gel), sodium bicarbonate (many generic products), sodium perborate.

Toothache and teething pain products

Drug category and indications for use

Local anesthetics, primarily benzocaine, are used topically to relieve sore throat and toothache pain, and gum pain associated with teething in infants.

Monograph ingredients

Benzocaine, benzyl alcohol, dyclonine, hexylrescorcinol, menthol, phenol, phenolate sodium, and salicyl alcohol (resorcinol) are used for toothache pain. Only benzocaine, phenol, and phenolate sodium are approved for relief of teething pain.[17]

Mode of action

Local anesthetics prevent and relieve pain by blocking nerve transmission from noxious stimuli that activate peripheral nerves.

Warnings and precautions

These products should not be used by anyone allergic to any ingredient. Products used for sore throat pain should not be used for more than 2 days; if symptom are not relieved or worsen, or if a headache or a fever develops, a physician should be consulted. If gum or toothache pain is not relieved, worsens, or lasts longer than 7 days, a dentist or physician should be consulted.[17]

Directions for use

Oral anesthetic/analgesic products used as ointments or gels for toothache pain by adults and children over 2 years of age should be rubbed along the gums of the affected tooth up to four times a day. Children between 2 and 12 years old should be supervised by a caregiver.

Benzocaine, phenol, and phenolate sodium are used for teething pain in infants over 4 months of age. Under that age, a physician should be consulted. Benzocaine may be rubbed on the gums up to four times a day. Fever and nasal congestion are not symptoms of teething and may be symptoms of some other condition, and a physician should be consulted.[11]

Products

Products for adult and children over 2 years of age: benzocaine (Zilactin B, Kanka), phenol (Campho-Phenique, Carmex), benzyl alcohol (Zilactin L and Kanka). Baby teething products: benzocaine (Baby Anbesol, Orajel Baby and Orajel Baby Nighttime).

Case study exercises

Case 1 A 52-year-old woman with narrow-angle glaucoma works at a computer everyday and complains of irritated, red eyes. She asks the pharmacist whether regular Visine or Visine A is better for her problem.

The pharmacist notes that the woman is taking a prescription drug to treat narrow-angle glaucoma. Both products the woman asked about contain a vasoconstrictor that should not be used when an individual has glaucoma. Vasoconstrictors are sympathomimetic amine drugs that constrict small blood vessels in the eye to reduce the redness, but they also cause the pupils of the eyes to dilate. This may worsen the glaucoma the woman has and impair her vision. The pharmacist recommends the use of an artificial tear solution or ointment. She should also take occasional breaks from looking at the computer monitor and be sure that she blinks more often to keep her eyes moist. If this doesn't solve her problem, she should consult her doctor.

Case 2 A young man has allergies to dust and molds. There is renovation construction going on in his apartment building and his eyes are itchy and watery.
This person would benefit most from an ophthalmic solution that contains an antihistamine. Two types of product are available, vasoconstrictor with an antihistamine (Naphcon A, Visine A, or Opcon A) or an ophthalmic solution containing only an antihistamine (Zaditor). The young man has no other medical condition, and could choose to use either product.

Case 3 A man asks the pharmacist to help him to select a disinfecting solution for contact lenses that his son wears because he doesn't know what to purchase.
The pharmacist asks the man what type of contact lenses his son wears, soft lenses or rigid gas permeable lenses. The man doesn't know. The pharmacist explains that she can't make any recommendation because each type of contact lens requires a different solution and they cannot be used interchangeably.

Case 4 A young woman who swims on the high school team asks for some type of product to get rid of the water in her ears.
The pharmacist recommends either Auro Ear or Swim Ear. Each product contains isopropyl alcohol in anhydrous glycerin and she should use four to five drops in each ear.

Case 5 The mother of a 7-year-old child asks the pharmacist for vitamins with fluoride.
The pharmacist tells the mother that vitamins or supplements with fluorides are prescription drugs and she should contact her dentist or physician. However, she could be sure that the toothpaste she buys is an anticaries (anticavity) product because it would contain fluoride. She should also purchase a topical fluoride rinse product like Phos-flur, Act or Listerine's Tooth Defense or Smart Rinse. The mother should be told that these products are to be swished around the teeth and then spat out. They are not intended to be swallowed.

Case 6 A young woman wants a mouth rinse that will help to reduce the build-up of plaque that she gets on her teeth.
The pharmacist discusses the need for thorough brushing and flossing of teeth as the best preventative for removing plaque rather than relying solely on a mouth rinse. A mouth rinse will be most effective if it is used after brushing the teeth. Suitable products are Listerine, Scope, Cepacol or Crest Pro-Health rinses.

Case 7 A 23-year-old woman who went to a tanning salon complains to the pharmacist that she thinks she has a cold sore, but she doesn't have a cold. She wants to know what to do.
The pharmacist explains that ultraviolet light from the tanning salon probably activated the herpes simplex virus that causes cold sores. There are two possible ways to treat her problem. The use of 10% docosanol (Abreva) applied topical five times a day could reduce the healing time for the cold sore. She could also apply topical oral anesthetics/external analgesics to relieve pain and discomfort. Products include benzocaine (Zilactin B or Anbesol), phenol (Carmex or Campho-Phenique), or benzyl alcohol (Zilactin L).

Case 8 The mother of an 11-month-old child wants to purchase a baby teething product but isn't sure how to use it.
The pharmacist explains that the solution or ointment should be rubbed along the gum where the tooth is going to erupt. If the product contains benzocaine, it may be used up to four times a day. Suitable products are Baby Anbesol, Orajel Baby and Orajel Baby Nighttime.

References

1. Ophthalmic drug products for over-the-counter human use; final monograph; final rule. *Fed Regist* 1988; 53: 7076–7093.
2. Ophthalmic drug products for over-the-counter human use; ophthalmic anti-infective drug products for over-the-counter human use. *Fed Regist* 1992; 57: 60416–60423.
3. Ophthalmic drug products for over-the-counter human use; amendment of final monograph. *Fed Regist* 2000; 65: 38426–38429.
4. *Zaditor Label.* www.zaditor.com/info/answers/drug-facts.jsp (accessed February 3, 2009).
5. *Contact Lens Solutions and Products.* Updated November 6, 2008. www.fda.gov/cder/contactlenses/solutions.html (accessed February 4, 2009).
6. Topical otic drug products for over-the-counter human use; final monograph: final rule. *Fed Regist* 1986; 51: 28656–28661.
7. Topical otic drug products for over-the-counter human use; products for drying water-clogged ears; amendment of monograph; lift of partial stay of effective date. *Fed Regist* 2000; 48902–48905.
8. Anticaries drug products for over-the-counter human use; final monograph. *Fed Regist* 1995; 60: 53474–52510.

9. *Toothbrushing*. www.ada.org/public/topics/cleaning_faq.asp (accessed February 4, 2009).
10. Oral health care drug products for over-the-counter human use; antigingivitis/antiplaques products; establishment of a monograph. *Fed Regist* 2003; 68: 32232–32287.
11. Oral health care products for over-the-counter human use: tentative final monograph; notice of proposed rulemaking. *Fed Regist* 1991; 56: 48302–48347.
12. Hirsh MS. Herpes simplex virus. In: Mandell GL *et al.* eds. *Principles and Practices of Infectious Diseases*, 4th edn. New York: Churchill Livingstone, 1995: 1336–1345.
13. *Docosanol*. www.fda.gov/cder/foi/nda/2000/20-941_Abreva.htm, (accessed February 7, 2009).
14. Orally administered drug products for the treatment of fever blisters for over-the-counter human use; final monograph. *Fed Regist* 1992; 57: 29166–29173.
15. Skin protection and external analgesic drug products for fever blister and cold sore treatment drug products. *Fed Regist* 1990; 55: 3362–3383.
16. Pope LE *et al.* The anti-herpes simplex virus activity of *n*-docosanol includes inhibition of the viral entry process. *Antiviral Res* 40: 1998; 85–94.

8

Topical dermatological products

The skin is the largest organ of the body and its main functions are to provide protection to the other organs and to regulate body temperature. It also has a cosmetic or esthetic purpose; it is the image that an individual first sees of another person and creates the first impression of that person. The FDA regulates products that affect the function and structure of the skin as drugs and those that affect its appearance as cosmetics, by the authority granted by the passage of the FD&C Act of 1938 and its amendments.

Labels for products that are cosmetics have major differences from labels of drugs. Products that are purely cosmetic have no active ingredients list, just a list of ingredients. All ingredients in the product are listed in the order of highest concentration of the ingredients first and the lowest concentrations last. The label does not contain the specific concentration of the ingredient, making the comparisons among products a nearly impossible task. Manufacturers may use either the chemical name or the trade name of the ingredient. Trade names do not provide a clear identity of the ingredient, making product comparisons even more difficult.[1]

Dermatological products that contain a drug and cosmetic ingredients must list the drug component as an active drug ingredient providing its approved drug name, the quantity of drug present, and any warnings or precautions. The cosmetic components are listed as inactive ingredients. Examples of this are many cosmetic skin moisturizers, which now contain a sunscreen. The sunscreen is an OTC drug approved by the FDA and must be listed as an active ingredient, and the remaining moisturizing components are listed as the inactive ingredients. Another example is hair shampoos. If the shampoo claims to eliminate or prevent dandruff, a drug claim, it must list the antidandruff ingredient as the active ingredient, and the other shampoo ingredients become inactive ingredients.

The skin is composed of two separate layers, the epidermis and the dermis. The epidermis has five separate layers, with the stratum germinativum, the basal layer, separating the epidermis from the dermis. Epithelial cells have a relatively uniform shape and high water content. As the cells grow upward toward the surface, they become more irregular in shape and lose moisture, becoming more flattened or packed together. The other layers of the skin are the stratum spinosum, the stratum granulosum, the stratum lucidum (a special band of tightly packed cells only found on the palms of the hands and soles of the feet), and the stratum corneum, the outermost layer.[2] The stratum spinosum contains melanocytes, which produce melanin when stimulated by the ultraviolet rays of sunlight to protect the skin.

The stratum corneum is a rather thin layer of keratinized cells (basically dead cells with the lowest water content, approximately 10 to 20%) forming a continuous, uniform layer that is continuously shed. These keratinized cells protect the layers of cells beneath by preventing the penetration of many compounds, especially those that are water soluble, to which the skin is exposed. The pH of the surface of the skin is slightly acidic, approximately 4.5 to 5.5, which prevents the growth of most microorganisms. Once the skin is damaged and this continuous layer of protection is broken, the risk of infection is greatly increased.

The dermis is a much thicker layer of cells, collagen, and elastin that separates the epidermis from the subcutaneous layer of tissue. It contains many vital structures, including nerves, the capillary network of the circulatory system, hair follicles, sebaceous glands, and sweat glands. The subcutaneous layer, hypodermis, consists of connective tissue, adipose tissues, and blood vessels and is responsible for providing nutrition to the layers above and for regulating body temperature.[2]

When the body temperature increases, the blood vessels dilate, and blood from the core of the body moves to the periphery or skin surface where cooling can occur. The sweat glands are innervated by the peripheral sympathetic nervous system, which stimulates the active secretion of water, causing heat loss by evaporation from the skin surface.

The moisture and lipid content of skin change with age and other conditions. Babies have a thinner epidermis with a higher water content and this allows greater absorption of many topical drugs. The epidermis becomes thicker in children and the secretion from the sebaceous glands increases during puberty, primarily as a result of increased hormone secretion, increasing the risk of acne in this age group.

Normal aging produces a great number of changes in the skin. The skin becomes thinner and loses moisture more readily, and there is a decrease in sebaceous gland and sweat gland secretions. These changes may produce dry skin (xerosis), one of the most common skin conditions in both men and women over the age of 65. The problem is exacerbated in women as they reach menopause because of the dramatic decrease in estrogen secretion; it occurs in men at a slightly older age as their testosterone levels decrease.[3]

Collagen and elastin deteriorate and wrinkles develop, primarily as a consequence of damage to the skin from environmental conditions (wind and sun), smoking, and other environmental or occupational chemicals, which may cause oxidation in skin cells. Skin damage also makes the skin more susceptible to flaking and cracking, causing a loss of continuity of the skin barrier and increasing susceptibility to infection.

There are disorders in skin cell turnover rates that cause dandruff, seborrhea, and psoriasis. This chapter discusses OTC drug therapy used to prevent or treat these conditions. This chapter also includes products used to treat dermatitis resulting from a variety of sources, insect bites and stings, and mild to moderate conditions causing itching, irritation, or pain to the skin, mucous membranes, or superficial muscles.

All of the products in this chapter are topical dermatological products and every product must bear a statement that indicates the product is for external use only.

Xerosis (dry skin)

When the water content of the epidermis falls below 10%, changes in the skin become very prominent, including chaffing, flaking, itching, redness (erythema), and roughness. As the skin becomes thinner and secretions from the sebaceous glands decrease, the permeability of the skin changes, allowing moisture from the lower layers of the skin to penetrate through the stratum corneum to the surface. Excessive bathing and harsh soaps remove lipids from the skin and exacerbate the problem.[3]

Bathing with tepid water rather than hot water and using super-fatted soaps such as glycerin soaps or nonsoap cleansers such as Aquanil Lotion or Cetaphil Lotion helps to prevent xerosis.

Environmental conditions of wind and low humidity increase loss of moisture. Xerosis is commonly referred to as alligator or lizard skin by individuals who have this problem because of the appearance of deep wrinkles.

Treatment of xerosis includes the use of skin protectants that have lipid characteristics to act as occlusive agents and prevent loss of moisture from the epidermis. Glycerin is generally considered to be a humectant type of skin protectant. It absorbs moisture and keeps it on the skin. Occlusive protectants are more effective in preventing loss of moisture but their greasy texture may be undesirable for some individuals. Most products used to moisturize the skin contain several different protective ingredients.[3]

Emollients and humectants (moisturizers)

Drug category and indications for use

Emollients and humectants are protective drugs applied to the epidermis to retard loss of moisture and to relieve symptoms associated with dry skin. They are used to protect chapped hands or lips, and to provide protection from the drying effects of wind and cold weather.[4]

Monograph ingredients

Skin protectants are used in treating numerous conditions depending on the specific concentration and product formulation. Most products contain more than one ingredient. The most commonly used protectants are beeswax, cocoa butter, dimethicone, glycerin, hard fat, lanolin, mineral oil, petrolatum, and white petrolatum. Table 8.1 lists the concentrations of each protectant that must be used to have it listed as an active ingredient in a drug product.[4] When the concentration of a protectant in a product is less than those in table 8.1, the label lists it as an inactive ingredient, not an active ingredient.

Mode of action

Emollients act as a barrier to prevent evaporation of moisture from the epidermal layers of the skin. The greater the lipid characteristic of the drug, the more effective it is as an occlusive agent. Emollients themselves contain no moisture.

Humectants are hygroscopic drugs that absorb water and hold it on the surface of the skin, allowing the epidermal keratin to become soft and supple. Glycerin is a true humectant.

Table 8.1 Protectants and concentrations required to be monograph or active ingredients for xerosis (dry skin): over-the-counter drug products and other topical dermatological products

Protectant	Monograph concentrations (%)
Cocoa butter	50–100
Cod liver oil	5–13.56
Colloidal oatmeal	> 0.007
Dimethicone	1–30
Glycerin	20–45
Hard fat	50–100
Lanolin	12.5–50
Mineral oil	50–100
Petrolatum	30–100
Topical starch	10–98
White petrolatum	30–100
Zinc acetate	0.1–2
Zinc carbonate	0.2–2
Zinc oxide	1–25

Product formulations include creams, ointments, gels, or lip balms, specifically for chapped lips.

Warnings and precautions

These products are intended for external use only and should not be used in or near the eyes. If the condition worsens or the product does not provide relief within 7 days, a physician should be consulted.[4]

Recommended use

Products intended for application to the skin should be applied at least twice a day. Products are most effective if applied after bathing. The skin should be patted dry and the protectant applied while the skin is still moist. Products intended as hand moisturizers should be applied as necessary. Products intended as lip protectants should be applied as necessary.[3,4]

Products

Beeswax (Burt's Bees Beeswax Lip Balm), dimethicone (Aveeno Skin Relief Moisturizing Cream, Aveeno Daily Moisturizing Lotion, Blistex Medicated Lip Balm, Chap Stick Overnight Lip Treatment, Natural Ice Medicated Lip Protectant), white petrolatum (Aveeno Lip Protectant, Vaseline Petroleum Jelly, Vaseline Lip Therapy, Chap Stick Lip Balm Original).

Popular moisturizing products that contain multiple protective ingredients include AmLactin, Eucerin, Keri Lotion, Alpha Keri, Jergens, Curel, Corn Huskers, Lubriderm, Moisturel, and Neutragena. Personal preference based on the texture or feel of the product on the skin is usually the deciding factor in choice of a product by most individuals who use skin protectant products.

Eczema (dermatitis)

Eczema is a general term used to describe an inflammatory condition of the skin that is characterized by redness, a rash, and/or itching. All of these symptoms may be considered to be some form of dermatitis. The most common form of eczema is *atopic dermatitis*. It has a genetic component and there is an increase in immunoglobulin E. It usually affects other members of the family, all of whom tend to have sensitive skin and other allergies, such as seasonal rhinitis (hay fever). Atopic individuals also tend to have a higher incidence of asthma.[5]

The incidence of atopic dermatitis is approximately 10 to 20% in children and decreases to less than 3% in adults. It is characterized by intense itchy, dry skin and may progress to papules or vesicles, with or without exudates, that occur primarily on the forehead, cheeks, chin, upper arms, wrists, ankles, and trunk of the body. Scratching may increase the risk of infection, and treatment includes the use of emollients (moisturizers) and antipruritic drugs. Oral antihistamines may be used to relieve the itching and topical corticosteroids are used because of their anti-inflammatory action.[5]

Other common skin problems include *allergic dermatitis*. The best treatment for these conditions is avoidance of the agent responsible for the dermatitis if it can be identified. Common allergens include soaps, detergents, fragrances, fabrics like wool, foods, drugs, metals like chromium or nickel (in jewelry), and plants, especially those in the *Toxicodendron* family (poison ivy, poison oak, poison sumac).

Irritant dermatitis results from continued contact of irritants on the skin; the most common causes are diaper rash and occupational exposure to chemicals. Symptoms include irritation, erythema, discomfort, and pain; the skin reaction may progress to breakdown of the skin, increasing susceptibility to infection. Treatment includes avoidance of the irritant: changing baby's diaper frequently and keeping the area clean and dry, or wearing protective clothing and/or gloves for occupational exposures. The use of skin protectants (discussed above) is the first line of treatment for these conditions, along with topical corticosteroids and antipruritic drugs.

Atopic dermatitis

Monograph drugs

Protectants
All protectants listed for xerosis in table 8.1 are approved for use in atopic dermatitis.

Rx–OTC switch drug: hydrocortisone
Hydrocortisone was initially introduced to the OTC market as a Rx–OTC switched drug in concentrations of 0.25 to 0.5%. The FDA added hydrocortisone to the External Analgesic Monograph and increased the permitted OTC concentration to 1%.

Drug category and indication for use
Topical hydrocortisone is a corticosteroid used to relieve the itch, redness and rash in eczema, psoriasis, insect bites and stings, and allergic skin reactions from soaps, detergents, cosmetics, jewelry, poison ivy, poison oak, and poison sumac.[6,7]

Mode of action
Hydrocortisone acts to suppress the immune system, reducing the symptoms associated with allergic reactions. It also prevents the inflammatory response and suppresses erythema and itching.

Warnings and precautions
Topical hydrocortisone is for external use only. It should not be used in the vagina or rectum. It may be used for itching on the skin area around the

vagina, but it should not be use if a vaginal discharge is present. It should not be used for external anal or genital itching in children under 12 years of age. Topical hydrocortisone should not be used in children under 2 years of age without consulting a physician. It should not be used for diaper rash without consulting a physician.

If the condition gets worse, if there is no relief in 7 days, or if the condition returns, a physician should be consulted.[6,7]

Recommended use
Hydrocortisone 0.25 or 1% may be applied to affected area three to four times a day by adults or children over 2 years of age.

Products
Hydrocortisone 1% (Cortaid and Cortizone10).

Irritant dermatitis: diaper rash

Diaper rash or diaper dermatitis has several causes, including excess moisture retention on the buttocks, perineum, lower abdomen and back and inner thighs and irritation from urine and/or feces. Changing the diaper frequently and use of protectants are recommended. If the skin becomes macerated and broken, infection is possible and a physician should be consulted.

Drug category and indications for use
Application of protectants to the affected area may prevent diaper rash and provide protection against wetness.[8]

Monograph ingredients
Cod liver oil (5 to 13.56%), lanolin (15.5%), mineral oil (50 to 100%), talc (45 to 100%), topical starch (10 to 98%), and zinc oxide (25 to 40%) are the only protectants recognized for diaper rash.[7,8] These drugs may be used alone or combined in a single product.

Mode of action
Topical protectants provide a physical barrier against wetness and irritants and prevent skin damage.

Warnings and precautions
If the diaper rash worsens or persists for longer than 7 days, or if it clears up but reoccurs in a few days, a physician should be consulted.

Cod liver oil is a source of vitamin A and D and no more than 10 000 units of vitamin A or 400 units of vitamin D (cholecalciferol) should be used in a 24 hour period.

Powdered topical starch should not be applied to broken skin and should not be used near the face to avoid inhalation.

Table 8.2 Selected popular diaper rash products containing protectants

Product[a]	Lanolin	Petrolatum	Cod liver oil (vitamins A and D)	Zinc oxide
A and D Original Ointment	M	M	I	
Aveeno Baby Soothing Relief				M
Balmex Extra Protective		M		
Boudreaux's Butt Paste		I		M
Desitin Original Ointment	I	I	I	M
Desitin Multi-Purpose	I	M	I	
Palmer's Bottom Butter		M	I	
Triple Paste	M	M		M

M, monograph concentrations; I, listed as inactive ingredients (concentration less than the required amount for monograph status).
[a]Products contain additional inactive ingredients.

Recommended use

The diaper area is cleaned and the product applied liberally with each diaper change, especially at bedtime.

Products

Table 8.2 lists popular diaper rash ointments or creams and lists the ingredients in each. Baby powder products include protectants but not in concentrations high enough to be classified as monograph ingredients. Talc is available in Johnson's Original Baby Powder, and corn starch is available in Johnson's Cornstarch Baby Powder and Burt's Bees Baby Powder.

Allergic contact dermatitis: poison ivy, poison oak, poison sumac

The best approach to allergic dermatitis is preventing the allergen from touching the skin or mucous membranes. The symptoms associated with allergic dermatitis include itching, erythema, rash, or blister formation. All of the protectants discussed earlier in this chapter will provide temporary relief for the symptoms associated with allergic contact dermatitis. Poison ivy, poison oak, and poison sumac are the most common plant causes of allergic dermatitis, and specific products have been developed for their treatment that usually include more than one monograph ingredient because of the intense itch that they cause.

These plants belong to the genus *Toxicodendron*, and they all produce an oleoresin, urushiol, that quickly and tenaciously binds to skin proteins (hence the names of urushiol-induced dermatitis and Toxicodendron dermatitis). All of these plants have green leaves that are in clusters of three, and they may have white, waxy-like berries. The leaves of poison ivy usually turn red in the fall. Poison ivy may act like a vine, wrapping itself on tree trunks. Herbicides are available that will kill the plants, but plants should not be burned because they may release oleoresin into the air, allowing for its further dispersion and increasing the risk of exposure. The oleoresin may remain on garden tools and clothing for months or years, causing re-exposure to individuals. All contaminated objects should be thoroughly cleaned. Pets may carry the resin on their fur and remain an additional source of exposure to those allergic to the oleoresin.[9]

Washing the contaminated skin within 5 to 10 minutes may remove the resin, but if more than an hour has elapsed, washing will not be effective. Several manufacturers make cleansing products that are not drug products for removing the oleoresin from the skin, but avoidance or wearing clothing and gloves that fully protects the skin is the best prevention.

Products promoted for removal of the oleoresin from the skin may contain surfacants (e.g. Zanfel Poison Ivy Wash and Cortaid Poison Ivy Care Toxin Removal Cloths) or may combine surfactants with microfine beads (e.g. IvyStat). The combination products act like very mild abrasives, causing exfoliation of the epidermis to eliminate the bound oleoresin. Most products recommend washing the contaminated skin as soon as possible, usually within a few hours of exposure. Products containing skin protectants, topical hydrocortisone, or external analgesics may be applied after their use.

Technu is also a product promoted for removal of oleoresin from the skin; it is a petroleum-based product, deodorized mineral spirits, and contains surfactants. However, it should not be used on skin if hydrocortisone products were used within the previous 3 days.[10]

Exposure of the skin to urushiol usually results in intense itching as the initial symptom, with erythema and a rash developing with a day or two. The intensity of rash depends on the amount of resin deposited on the skin. If an individual just brushed by the plant, the erythema and rash forms a linear or jagged path. Intense exposure produces a continuous, redden patch on the skin. The rash progresses to form papules, bullae, and vesicles that fill with fluid, but the fluid does not contain resin and is not contagious, contrary to popular belief. How quickly the rash forms depends on the amount of resin on the skin. The ruptured vesicles form a crust and complete healing may take 2 or 3 weeks.[9]

Self-care may be appropriate if the exposed area is relatively small, but widespread exposure is best treated by oral corticosteroids prescribed by a physician. Exposure around the eyes, the mucous membranes of the nose and mouth, or the genitals warrants consultation with a physician. Scratching the intense itch increases the risk of infection; if a fever develops or pus forms in the blisters, a physician must be consulted.[9]

Prevention of urushiol exposure: bentoquatum

Drug category and directions for use

Bentoquatum, an inert, silicate clay (quaternium-18 bentonite), is applied to the skin to prevent exposure to urushiol oleoresin.

FDA approved new drug application

Bentoquatum 5%.

Mode of action

Topical application of bentoquatum to the skin creates a physical barrier. The oleoresin adheres to the clay, protecting the skin from direct contact with the allergen.[11]

Warnings and precautions

Bentoquatum should not be used on broken skin or open rash or in children under 6 years of age. The product should be shaken well before use.[12]

Recommended use

Bentoquatum is applied topically to the exposed area of skin 15 minutes before risk of exposure to plants and reapplied every 4 hours, or sooner if sweating profusely.[12]

Product

Bentoquatum 5% (Ivy Block).

Treatment of urushiol exposure: protectants

Several different pharmacological agents are used to treat the rash and itch associated with poison ivy. Colloidal oatmeal and sodium bicarbonate are skin protectants that soothe the irritated and erythematous skin. Itching is an irritating, cutaneous sensation than causes an individual to scratch. Topical analgesics have local anesthetic activity, blocking the nerves that are responsible for producing the itching sensation. Combinations of protectants and external analgesics are found in nearly all products for treating poison ivy.[13]

Drug category and indications for use

Skin protectants provide temporary relief from minor irritation and itching caused by poison ivy, poison oak, or poison sumac.

Monograph ingredients

Colloidal oatmeal and sodium bicarbonate (1 to 100%) are the most frequently used skin protectives. Calamine is frequently used. It contains zinc oxide with 1% or less of ferric oxide to produce a pink tint to lotions, creams, or ointments; colorless calamine products have no ferric oxide.[4]

Mode of action

Skin protectants prevent drying and itching of the skin from harmful stimuli.

Warnings and precautions
All products are for external use only.

Colloidal oatmeal contains the following warnings.[13] 'Use a mat in the tub or shower to prevent slipping when use as a soaking preparation; soaking too long may cause excessive drying of the skin; stir any colloidal oatmeal that may settle on the bottom of the tub; use only once and discard solution.'

Recommended use
Adults and children over 2 years of age should soak the affect areas for 15 to 30 minutes when colloidal oatmeal is used. The area should be patted dry, and the process may be repeated as needed or as directed by a physician. Colloidal oatmeal used as a wet compress should be applied for 15 to 30 minutes and may be repeated as needed. A freshly prepared compress should be prepared each time it is needed.

Sodium bicarbonate may be used by adults and children over 2 years of age as a paste and applied to the affected area as needed or directed by a physician. If it is to be used as a soak, 1 to 2 cupfuls should be dissolved in warm water and the individual should soak the affected area for 15 to 30 minutes and the area should be patted dry. It should only be used once and a fresh solution should be prepared each time it is needed.[13]

Treatment of urushiol exposure: external analgesics

Drug category and indications for use
External analgesics may temporarily relieve itch and discomfort caused by skin rashes, including those from poison ivy, poison oak, poison sumac, insect bites and stings, and minor skin irritations.

Monograph ingredients
Diphenhydramine is the antihistamine used in most topical analgesic products.

Local anesthetics drugs include benzyl alcohol, phenol, phenolate sodium, benzocaine, dibucaine, lidocaine, and proxamine.[4,13]

Mode of action
The FDA definition of topical external analgesics includes topical antihistamines and topical local anesthetics. Topical antihistamines prevent the histamine produced by the allergic reaction from binding to cutaneous receptors, thus preventing or reducing redness and itching. Topical anesthetics affect the cutaneous nerves in the skin, blocking transmission of stimuli that cause itching and pain.

Warnings and precautions
Diphenhydramine should not be used over a large area of the skin and it should not be used when other topical or oral products containing diphenhydramine are used. It should not be used to treat itching and discomfort

Table 8.3 Monograph drug products for treating symptoms of poison ivy, poison oak and poison sumac, and insect bites

Product	Protectant	External analgesic
Aveeno Anti Itch Cream and Lotion	Colloidal oatmeal	Proxamine
Benadryl Itch Stopping Cream, Spray	Zinc acetate	Diphenhydramine
Calamine Lotion	Calamine (zinc oxide)	
Caladryl Clear Lotion	Zinc acetate	Diphenhydramine
Calagel Anti Itch Lotion	Zinc acetate	Diphenhydramine
Gold Bond Medicated Itch Relief		Proxamine
Ivarest Anti-Itch Cream	Calamine (zinc oxide)	Dephenhydramine
Itch-X Spray and Gel		Benzyl alcohol and pramoxine
Itch-X Anti-Itch Lotion		Hydrocortisone
Sarna Original Anti Itch Lotion		Camphor and menthol

associated with measles or chickenpox without consulting a physician. Both conditions may produce a rash over the entire body, increasing the risk of toxicity. There have been reports of confusion and psychosis in children from excess absorption of diphenhydramine.[14] Oral products containing diphenhydramine include those used for allergies, coughs, colds, sinus relief, motion sickness, and sedatives.

Local anesthetics should not be used if the individual has an allergy toward the specific ingredient, and lidocaine is not recommended for children under 2 years of age.[4,13]

If itching and discomfort are not relieved, or worsen within 7 days, a physician should be contacted.

Recommended dose

Topical products for poison ivy, poison oak, and poison sumac may be used three or four times a day as needed.

Products

Most products for poison ivy, poison oak and poison sumac contain a combination of external analgesics and skin protectants (table 8.3).

Insect bites and stings

Arthropods, a phylum of invertebrate animals that includes insects, commonly bite or sting humans and produce a burning, stinging sensation immediately or within a brief period of time; the area around the bite or sting becomes swollen, red, and itchy. The most serious effect an individual can experience is an anaphylactic allergic reaction, which may cause death through acute hypotension, circulatory collapse, bronchoconstriction, and respiratory arrest. These sensitive individuals should have a prescription for an epinephrine pen that they should carry at all times. The most common stinging arthropods are bumblebees, honey bees, yellow jackets, hornets, wasps, and scorpions. Bees leave their stinger in the skin and it should be removed carefully.

Ants, bed bugs, chiggers, fleas, black flies, gnats, lice, mosquitoes, scabies, spiders, and ticks are the most common biting arthropods. Ticks and mosquitoes are of special concern because they may transmit diseases.

Ticks, especially ticks whose main host are deer, transmit several serious diseases, the most common being Lyme disease and Rocky Mountain spotted fever. Ticks are parasites that remain on the skin and should be carefully removed by gently grasping the tick with forceps or tweezers and tugging until it is released from the skin. It should be kept for proper identification; deer ticks are much smaller than other ticks.

Mosquitoes are also common carriers of disease, and are responsible primarily for West Nile virus in the USA. Chiggers and scabies are parasitic mites that remain on the skin; their bites and secretions cause intense itching, inflammation, and skin irritation. Scabies burrow under the skin and may require physician treatment for their eradication.

Insect repellants

Prevention is the best solution to arthropod bites and stings. Avoid the use of perfumes or products that may attract arthropods. When going outdoors, especially in high grass or wooded areas, wear tight fitting clothing that is not brightly colored and covers as much of the skin as possible. Exposed skin surfaces may be protected by the application of topical insect repellents. The Environmental Protection Agency (EPA) regulates insect repellents.

EPA approved chemicals for human use

DEET (N,N-diethyl-m-toluamide), picaridin (KBR 3023 or 2-(2-hydroxyethyl)-1-piperidinecarboxylic acid 1-methylpropyl ester) and oil of lemon eucalyptus (PMD or para-menthane-3,8-diol) are approved for use on both human skin and clothing. These chemicals are effective against the most common arthropods, including flies, gnats, mosquitoes, and ticks.[15]

Mode of action
Insect repellents interfere with pheromone detection used by the insect to locate its prey.

Warnings and precautions for all products

Products should be applied only to exposed skin or clothing, and not on underclothing. Repellents should not be used on skin that has cuts, wounds, or is burned or irritated. They should be used sparingly around the eyes and mucous membranes of the nose and mouth. Application to the face is by spraying the product on the hands and then applying to the face, not by directly spraying the face with an aerosol. Adults should apply insect repellents for children and not allow them to handle products.[16]

Treated skin should be washed with soap and water when returning indoors. All clothing should also be washed before it is worn again. If the product causes skin irritation or a rash, it should be washed off immediately with soap and water. If product is ingested, the local poison control center should be called. The container of the product should be taken if a visit to the physician's office or the emergency center is needed. Empty containers should be disposed of properly and the container not reused.[16]

DEET has an odor and a greasy feel and may stain clothes. It should not be applied on or near fabrics containing acetates, rayon, spandex or other synthetic materials (excluding nylon), furniture, plastics, watch crystals, leather, or painted or varnished surfaces, including cars.

Warnings specifically for DEET. 'Excessive application may cause ataxia, confusion, blurred vision, and seizures. The higher the concentration of DEET applied to the skin, and the greater the area of application on the skin, the greater the risk of adverse effects. Do not use in children under 2 years of age without consulting a physician.'

Recommended use

DEET should be applied to exposed skin according to the EPA directions and may be re-applied if the insects begin to bite. DEET should not be used in children under 2 years of age without consulting a physician. The American Academy of Pediatrics does not recommend the use of DEET on infants younger than 2 months of age.[17] DEET should be used in concentrations less than 10% for children under 12 years of age. Adults may use concentrations of DEET as high as 100%. As the concentration of DEET applied to the skin increases, it provides a longer duration of protection.

Picaridin has fewer adverse effects and is preferred for use on children. It is nearly as effective as DEET against most insects. Effective concentrations range from 5 to 20%. It should be applied to exposed skin surfaces and may be re-applied if the insects begin to bite.[15]

Oil of lemon eucalyptus is effective against mosquitoes and ticks but it is not as effective as DEET or picaridin. It should be applied to exposed skin in concentrations of 30 to 40%. Oil of lemon eucalyptus is not recommended for use in children under 3 years of age.[15]

Products
DEET (Off! Deep Woods Sportsman, Off! Skintastic, Off! Deep Woods Insect Repellent, Off! Deep Woods Towelettes, Ben's Tick and Insect Repellent, and Ultrathon), picaridin (Cutter Advanced Insect Repellent and Natrapel 8 Hour DEET Free), oil of lemon eucalyptus (Repel Plant Based Lemon Eucalyptus Insect Repellent).

Insect bite and sting treatment

Oral antihistamines (Chapter 4) are also effective in relieving itch and inflammation associated with insect bites and stings. All arthropod bites and sites may be treated with topical hydrocortisone and external analgesics (antipruritics and local anesthetics, as discussed earlier in this chapter) used as single agents or combination products. The products listed in table 8.3 are also approved by the FDA for relief of itching and skin irritation from insect bites. Counterirritants are also used for treating insect bites and stings, either alone or combined with a protectant, an antipruritic, or a local anesthetic.

Drug category and indications for use
Counterirritants are used for the temporary relief of pain and itching caused by minor aches and pains.

Monograph ingredients
Allyl isothiocynate (0.05 to 5%), ammonia water (1 to 2.5%), camphor (3 to 11%), capsaicin (0.025 to 0.05%), histamine (0.025 to 0.1%), menthol (1.25 to 16%), methyl nicotinate (0.25 to 1%), methyl salicylate (10 to 60%), and turpentine oil (6 to 50%) are monograph counterirritants.[18]

Mode of action
Counterirritants are external analgesics that stimulate cutaneous sensory nerves for the purpose of relieving pain in deeper layers of the skin.[18]

Warnings and precautions
Counterirritants are for external use only and should not be used around the eyes, on wounds or damaged skin. The affected area should not be covered or bandaged. If the condition worsens or does not improve in 7 days, a physician should be consulted.

Recommended use
Counterirritants are applied to the affected area three to four times a day. They should not be used in children under 2 years of age without consulting a physician.

Products
Table 8.4 lists the external analgesic products available to treat insect bites and stings.

Table 8.4 Products containing external analgesic monograph ingredients for insect bites and stings

Product	Counterirritant	Local anesthetic	Protectant
After Bite Fast Itch Eraser			Sodium bicarbonate
After Bite	Ammonia		
Burt's Bees Bug Bite Relief	Camphor and menthol		
Mitigator Sting and Bite Scrub			Sodium bicarbonate
Sting Eze		Benzocaine	
Swab Plus Pre-filled Swabs		Benzocaine	

Pediculosis (lice infestations)

Lice are blood-sucking parasites that infest the head, body, or pubic area and are the only organisms amenable to self-treatment. They can cause intense itching and rashes. Head lice are the most common infestation problem in the USA and occur predominately in children. Female lice lay their eggs, commonly called nits, on the hair shaft near the scalp. The nits are bound to the hair by chitin and may be removed by combing with a fine-toothed comb or washing with medicated shampoos. The nits normally hatch in 7 to 10 days and the life cycle is repeated if the lice are not eradicated. Head lice are spread from one person to another by using objects that are contaminated, such as sharing combs, brushes, hats, or pillows.

Body lice occur less frequently and tend to inhabit clothing that is worn close to the skin. The lice feed off blood in the skin and eradication involves improving personal hygiene by bathing more frequently and washing contaminated clothing more frequently in hot water. Wearing contaminated clothing is the usual method for transmitting body lice from one person to another.

Pubic lice (crabs) physically resemble crabs and infest hair in the pubic area. Spread of pubic lice is usually through sexual contact. Underwear or other contaminated clothing should be washed in hot water and dried using the hot cycle for 20 minutes.

Treatment of lice includes the use of pediculicides and physical removal of nits by combing. Inanimate objects should be washed in hot water and dried for 20 minutes using the hot cycle in a dryer. Objects that cannot be cleansed in this manner may be dry-cleaned or stored in a plastic bag for 2 weeks. Adult lice may only survive for a couple of days without feeding, but the nits, if present, may not hatch for up to 10 days. The monograph recommends storage of the items for 2 weeks.[19]

There is a concern that resistance to the OTC products may have developed in lice. If all directions are not carefully followed and the treatment is not repeated in 7 to 10 days, reinfestation may occur. It is also possible that some type of genetic change may have occurred in lice, but this has not been clearly established. If lice remain after a second treatment, referral to a physician is necessary. Antibiotics or prescription pediculicides may be necessary to successfully treat the individual.

Monograph drugs

Drug category and indications for use
OTC pediculicide, pyrethrum extract, refers only to treatment for lice and includes head lice, body lice, and pubic lice.[20]

Monograph ingredients
Pyrethrum extract, formerly known as pyrethrins, combined with piperonyl butoxide is the only monograph drug.

Mode of action
Pyrethrum extract is derived from chrysanthemums and is absorbed by the lice, causing paralysis of the nervous system and death. These compounds are not absorbed by humans. Piperonyl butoxide is combined with pyrethrins because it inhibits the normal oxidative enzymes in lice from metabolizing pyrethrins to inactive compounds.[19]

Warnings and precautions
Pyrethrum extract should not be used near the eyes, on the eyebrows or eyelashes, or in the nose, mouth, or vagina. Pyrethrum extract should not be used without consulting a physician by anyone allergic to ragweed or chrysanthemums, because they may have difficulty breathing or an asthma attack. If breathing becomes difficult, or if irritation of the skin or eyes occurs, the product should be washed off and a physician consulted.

Recommended use
Products used as shampoos are applied to dry hair and remain on the hair for 10 minutes before being lathered with warm water to wash the hair. The hair is towel dried and any tangles combed out. A fine-toothed comb is then used to remove nits that remain on the hair shaft near the scalp. The hair should be treated again in 7 to 10 days. This product should not be used in children under 2 years of age without consulting a physician.[19]

Products
Pyrethrum extract with pipronyl butoxide (RID Shampoo and Pronto Lice Killing Mousse Shampoo).

New drug application: permethrin

Drug category and indications for use
An OTC pediculicide refers only to treatment for lice and includes head lice, body lice, and pubic lice.

Mode of action
Permethrin is a synthetic pyrethrin absorbed by lice that paralyses the nervous system, resulting in death.

Warnings and precautions
Permethrin should not be used near the eyes, on the eyebrows or eyelashes, or in the nose, mouth or vagina. Permethrin should not be used without consulting a physician by anyone allergic to ragweed. (Although permethrin is not derived from chrysanthemums, it is chemically related to natural pyrethrum and the individual may experience a sensitivity reaction.) Stop using permethrin if it causes a rash on the skin or scalp.[21]

Recommended use
The hair is washed with any shampoo that does not contain a conditioner and towel dried so it remains damp before applying the product. The product is kept on the hair for 10 minutes before rinsing with warm water and towel drying. Once tangles have been combed from hair, a fine-toothed comb is used to remove nits. A second treatment may be applied in 7 or more days if live lice remain. Permethrin should not be used in children under 2 months of age.[21]

Product
Permethrin (Nix).

Alternative therapy

Parents who do not want to use chemicals on their children have several other choices available for treating head lice. Products that moisten and add lubrication to the hair are available to make combing the nits from the hair easier. LiceMD contains dimethicone, and RID Egg & Nit Comb-Out Gel contains glycerin and cellulose derivatives. These products are not pediculicides. They are applied to the hair before combing with a fine-toothed comb and then washing the hair with warm water.[22]

Homeopathic pediculicide

Licefreee! is a homeopathic product that contains sodium chloride. The product forms a thick, gel that immobilizes the lice until they die. This product may create a hypertonic condition that affects the lice, but there is no explanation provided for its mechanism of action in the company's literature.[23]

The product is applied to dry hair and then covered with a plastic cap (shower cap), which is included with the product. The product is kept on the hair for at least 60 minutes and then the hair is washed with warm water. After towel drying and combing out tangles, the hair is combed with a fine-toothed comb. The treatment may be repeated in 7 to 10 days. Since most cases of head lice are in children, it may be difficult to persuade them to keep a wet gel on their head for 60 minutes, and this may limit the potential usefulness of this product.

Musculoskeletal pain

Mild to moderate pain and discomfort affecting the muscles, ligaments, tendons, and joints may occur after repetitive use or after minor injury and are frequently treated with topical analgesics. Osteoarthritis joint pain is frequently treated with topical analgesics. OTC oral analgesics (Chapter 5) may be successful in relieving pain for many individuals, but many others prefer to treat localized musculoskeletal problems by applying an external analgesic to the affected area.

The counterirritant drugs that were discussed earlier in this chapter are the drugs of choice for topical pain relief. The use of a cold or hot compress is useful in mitigating musculoskeletal pain. When a minor injury, such as twisting an ankle or knee, occurs, the body responds by increasing the blood supply to the area and inflammatory mediators are released, which may cause swelling and inflammation. This response may be reduced by resting the affected area, applications of ice, wrapping the injury with an elastic-type bandage to produce compression, and elevation of the injured area if possible to reduce swelling. The acronym RICE describes this process.

Application of a cold compress, ice, or cold packs to the area will reduce the inflammatory response, providing temporary relief of pain. Cold applications should last for approximately 10 or 15 minutes and may be used three or four times within the first 24 hours after the injury.

There are products available containing chemicals that produce an endothermic reaction, producing a cold compress for immediate use. These products can be used only one time. Reusable gel packs that are stored before use in a freezer or ice may be used. If ice is used, it should not be placed on bare skin. It may be placed in an ice bag or a plastic bag and wrapped in a towel before applying it to the skin.

There are also products available containing chemicals that produce an exothermic reaction, providing an immediate source of heat when needed. Warm compresses, heating pads, moist steam packs, reusable gel packs, and heat wraps (ThermaCare Heat Wraps) or patches are all available as sources of heat. Heat wraps may only be used only once and are discarded. After 24 hours, the application of heat may be more appropriate than cold to relieve discomfort. Heat should never be applied to the skin if a counterirritant has been used on the skin because it will increase absorption of the counterirritant and may damage the skin.

Some counterirritant drugs such as camphor and menthol may cause a feeling of coolness of the skin, while others like methyl salicylate (oil of wintergreen) cause warmth. Capsaicin and trolamine (triethanolamine salicylate) have no noticeable effect on the skin's temperature. Most products used as topical analgesics contain more than one counterirritant and may contain a local anesthetic and/or a protectant.

Drug category and indications for use

Counterirritants are topical external analgesics that may be used for the temporary relief of minor aches and pains of muscles and joints caused by a simple backache, lumbago (an old term referring to lower back pain), arthritis, neuralgia, strains, bruises, and sprains.[18]

Monograph counterirritants

Camphor, capsaicin, menthol, and methyl salicylate are monograph drugs.

Mode of action

Counterirritants stimulate cutaneous sensory nerve fibers by causing mild irritation or inflammation and in doing so mask the pain in the deeper layer of the tissue that was caused by the injury or other noxious stimuli.[18]

Menthol and camphor produce a cooling sensation on the skin initially that is followed by a feeling of warmth, which may be mediated by inhibition of cutaneous catecholamines.[24]

Capsaicin, a compound derived from peppers, causes the depletion of substance P, a neuropeptide present in peripheral sensory nerve fibers. This occurs only with repeated application for 7 to 14 days. Capsaicin causes no feelings of either coolness or warmth.[24]

Methyl salicylate produces a feeling of warmth on the skin and is presumed to act by inhibiting local prostaglandins that sensitize nerve receptors to pain.[18] Trolamine may produce a similar effect because it is also a salicylate. However, the FDA has not issued a final ruling on the efficacy of trolamine at this time, and it appears in several products.

Warnings and precautions

These products are for external use only and should not be used around the eyes or on mucous membranes. If the condition worsens or persists for more than 7 days, a physician should be consulted. The products should not be applied to wounds or damaged skin and the treated area should not be bandaged or covered.[18]

Recommended dose

These products are applied to the affected area three to four times a day. They should not be used for children under 2 years of age without consulting a physician.

Table 8.5 Products containing monograph-listed counterirritant combinations (external analgesics) for musculoskeletal pain and osteoarthritis

Product	Camphor	Menthol	Methyl salicylate	Capsaisin
Banalag	Yes	Yes	Yes	
Ben Gay Pain Relieving Cream	Yes	Yes	Yes	
Biofreeze Roll on	Yes	Yes		
Pain Bust-R		Yes	Yes	
Salonpas Pain Patch	Yes	Yes	Yes	Yes
Salonpas Gel Patch		Yes		Yes
Salonpas Arthritis Patch		Yes	Yes	
Salonpas Pain Relief Patch-Ultra Thin		Yes	Yes	
Thera-Gesic		Yes	Yes	
Tiger Balm and Tiger Balm Arthritis	Yes	Yes		
Zen Sports Balm	Yes	Yes	Yes	

Products

Menthol (Absorbine Jr Spray, Aspercreme Heat Pain Relieving Gel, Ben Gay Gel and Patch, Biofreeze Gel and Spray, Icy Hot Lotion and Patch, Mineral Ice and Ultra Blue), capsaicin (Capzasin-P and Zostrix); trolamine (Myoflex, Sportscreme, and Mobisyl). Table 8.5 contains the list of topical counterirritants products that are combinations and their monograph ingredients.

Hemorrhoids

Hemorrhoids, a common anorectal condition, are frequently treated with OTC products if there is no rectal bleeding. Hemorrhoids are swollen veins in the anorectal area. These veins have thin walls and become dilated and bleed. Hemorrhoids are either internal, above the anorectal line covered with mucous membranes that lack pain receptors, or external, below the anorectal line and covered with epithelial skin that has pain receptors. The anorectal line is the area where the upper anal canal merges with the rectum.[25,26] A commonly used term used to describe hemorrhoids is piles.

Symptoms associated with hemorrhoids include irritation, itching, discomfort, pain, and rectal bleeding, occurring most frequently during bowel movements. If rectal bleeding occurs, it is usually bright red, and further diagnosis and treatment require consultation with a physician. If the diagnosis of hemorrhoids was made previously, a physician should again be consulted because some other condition may now be present. Many serious conditions may cause rectally bleeding, including colon cancer, cirrhosis of the liver, obstructions, fissures, and tumors.

The cause of hemorrhoids in many individuals may be unknown, but certain situations are associated with the development of hemorrhoids, such as excessive straining during defecation, frequent diarrhea, and pregnancy. The weight of the fetus on the blood vessels in the membranes lining the floor of the pelvis and the pressures exerted during normal vaginal delivery of the baby may cause hemorrhoids in women. Often, after delivery, the condition may resolve or it could return at some later stage of life.[25]

Individuals should be take measures to prevent constipation by having some bulk or fiber in their diets, drinking plenty of fluids, and by taking a stool softener. The anal area should be carefully cleansed after a bowel movement, and should be patted dry, not vigorously rubbed. Premoistened anorectal wipes with or without medication or baby wipes can be used for cleansing the area. Application of topical OTC astringents, external analgesics, skin protectants, keratolytics, and vasoconstrictor drugs approved by the FDA are available for self-treatment of hemorrhoids. External analgesics and skin protectants discussed previously in this chapter are used to treat hemorrhoids.

Dosage formulations for anorectal products include cream, ointments, medicated wipes or pads for cleansing, and suppositories. Some products may be inserted intrarectally with an applicator or a 'hemorrhoid pipe'.

Astringents

Drug category and indications of use
Astringents provide a coagulant effect on skin or mucous membranes to provide relief from itching and discomfort associated with hemorrhoids and aids in protecting irritated anorectal areas.

Monograph ingredients
Calamine (5 to 25%), witch hazel (10 to 50%), formerly Hamamelis water, and zinc oxide (5 to 25%) are monograph astringents. Note that calamine and zinc oxide are also classified as skin protectants.

Mode of action
Astringents reduce the amount of mucus and other secretions that may irritate and inflame the affected area.[26,27]

Warnings and precautions
If the condition worsens or does not improve within 7 days, the individual should consult a physician. If bleeding occurs, a physician should be consulted promptly.

Recommended use

The individual should apply these products to the affected area after proper cleansing. These products should not be used on children less than 12 years of age.

Products

Calamine, witch hazel and zinc oxide are available as single products from many generic manufacturers. Table 8.6 lists combination products including these ingredients when they are used for hemorrhoid relief.

Table 8.6 Hemorrhoidal relief products that contain a combination of monograph astringents, external analgesics, protectants or vasoconstrictors

Product	Astringent	External analgesic	Protectant	Vasoconstrictor	Use[a]
Americaine Ointment		Benzocaine			E
Lanacane		Hydrocortisone			E
Nupercainal Ointment		Dibucaine			E
Preparation H Anti-itch		Hydrocortisone			E
Preparation H Cream, Maximum Strength		Pramoxine	Glycerin, petrolatum, shark liver oil	Phenylephrine	E
Preparation H suppository			Cocoa butter, shark liver oil	Phenylephrine	I
Preparation H ointment	Witch hazel		Mineral oil, petrolatum, shark liver oil	Phenylephrine	I and E
Preparation H Wipes	Witch hazel				E
Tronolane Cream		Pramoxine	Zinc oxide		I and E
Tronolane Suppository			Hard fat	Phenylephrine	I
Tucks pads	Witch hazel				E
Tucks Anti-itch Ointment		Hydrocortisone			E
Tucks Oint-ment (Anusol)		Pramoxine	Mineral oil, zinc oxide		E

[a] Use for internal (I) or external (E) hemorrhoids.

Keratolytics

Drug category and indications for use
Keratolytics debride surface cells of the epidermis to relieve the itching and discomfort associated with hemorrhoids.

Monograph ingredients
Alcloxa (0.2 to 2%) and resorcinol (1 to 3%) are the only kertolytics considered mild enough in their action to be used on the anorectal tissues.

Mode of action
Keratolytics act on keratin to loosen its attachment to epidermal cells so that the cells slough off.[26]

Warnings and precautions
If the individual's condition worsens or does not improve within 7 days, a physician should be consulted. If bleeding occurs, a physician should be consulted promptly. These products should not be used in the rectum.

Products
There are no keratolytic drugs available in the most popular anorectal products sold in the USA at this time, but they may appear in store or generic brands.

Vasoconstrictors

Drug category and indications for use
Vasoconstrictors are used to temporarily relieve the swelling of hemorrhoids.

Monograph ingredients
Epinephrine (0.005 to 0.01%), ephedrine (0.1 to 1.25%), and phenylephrine (0.25%) are vasoconstrictor drugs.

Mode of action
Vasoconstrictors are drugs that act on the alpha-adrenoceptors in the smooth muscle of blood vessel walls to shrink or constrict the vasodilated blood vessels.

Warnings and precautions
Individuals who have heart disease, high blood pressure, thyroid disease, diabetes, or difficulty in urination because of enlargement of the prostate gland should not use these products without consulting a physician. If an individual is taking drugs for high blood pressure or depression, a physician should be consulted before using these products.[26,27]

Ephedrine may cause insomnia, nervousness, nausea, loss of appetite, and tremor. The individual should consult a physician if these symptoms occur.[26,27]

Recommended dose
The products are applied to the affected area up to four times a day.

Products
See table 8.6.

Antiperspirants

The purpose of the eccrine sweat glands in the dermal layer of the skin is to provide a means of controlling body temperature. When conditions result in the core body temperature rising, there is an increase in secretions from the sweat glands. As the sweat evaporates from the skin, it causes cooling. Some individuals may have overactive sweat glands, while others perceive the appearance of any moisture under the arms as an embarrassment.

The FDA has approved certain salts of aluminum, which are astringents, as antiperspirants. Most individuals use antiperspirants daily, and these products have a minimum of adverse affects, the most common being skin irritation.

Drug category and indications for use
Antiperspirants are used to prevent or reduce the amount of sweat.[28]

Monograph ingredients
Aluminum chloride, aluminum chlorohydrate, aluminum chlorohydrex salts, and aluminum zirconium chlorohydrate salts are monograph antiperspirants. There are a total of 18 different aluminum salts approved in the monograph.[28]

Mode of action
Astringents precipitate (shrink or constrict) proteins within the sweat gland to reduce, lessen, or decrease secretions.

Warnings and precautions
Antiperspirants should not be applied on broken skin. If skin irritation or a rash occurs, use of the the product should stop. If the irritation or rash does not improve, the individual should contact a physician. Those with kidney disease should consult a physician before using these products. Users of spray products should avoid inhalation or contact with the eyes.

A popular internet myth links use of antiperspirants with breast cancer. A study published in the *Journal of the National Cancer Institute*[29] showed no such relationship and has been supported by a more recent study.[30]

Recommended use
The antiperspirant is applied topically to the underarms only. Products that reduced sweating by 20% may claim a 24 hour effect; products that reduce sweating by 30% may claim extra-effective protection.[28]

Products

All popular antiperspirants are aluminum salts in varying concentrations and may or may not contain a fragrance and are formulated for men or women. Products labeled as deodorants only are cosmetics not drugs.

Sunscreens

Many of the changes in the skin that are attributed to aging, especially in the epidermal layers, are really effects from damage caused by ultraviolet rays in sunlight (photoaging). Sun damage includes sunburn, photoaging, actinic keratoses, and skin cancer.

Ultraviolet in sunlight is divided into three categories depending on wavelength: UVA is 320–400 nanometers (nm), UVB 290–320 nm, and UVC 200–290 nm. There are two subdivisions of UVA: UVA-1 is 340–400 nm (long UVA) and UVA-2 is 320–340 nm (short UVA). The earth's natural ozone layer absorbs UVC. Artificially produced UVC is used for germicidal purposes in sterilizing inanimate objects.[31]

UVB is responsible for most of the damage referred to as sunburn, causing erythema or reddening and blistering. UVB strikes the earth primarily between 10:00 a.m. and 2:00 p.m. when the USA is using standard time. It is able to penetrate cloud cover and water and is reflected off water, snow, and sand. The best protection against exposure is to remain indoors or in the shade during this time period, or to cover the skin with clothing or sun-protective drugs.

The monograph sunscreens have a different degree of effectiveness in protecting the epidermis against ultraviolet light, and they are primarily effective against UVB. The FDA developed a method to describe the relative effectiveness of sunscreens to provide people with a tool to help them to decide which product would provide the degree of protection they need. The sun protection factor (SPF) is determined by using a standard source of ultraviolet light and exposing protected skin (skin with sunscreen applied) and unprotected skin to produce the same amount of erythema (redness) on the skin. The amount of energy required to produce erythema in protected skin divided by the energy required to produce erythema in unprotected skin determines the SPF value.[31]

A rating of SPF 4 provides the least amount of protection and is recommended for use primarily for individuals who have a high concentration of melanin in the skin. A product that has an SPF of 8 means that it takes twice as long to produce the same amount of skin damage, or it provides twice the protection as a product with SPF 4. The maximum SPF value has been increased from SPF 30+ to SPF 50+.[32]

Melanin is a pigment produced in the skin in response to exposure to sunlight to protect the skin from further damage, and is responsible for 'tanning' of the skin. Individuals who have fair skin have less melanin, especially if they are of Celtic origin, and should use products with SPF 30+ or higher for protection. Cosmetic products that produce an artificial tan on the skin provide no sun protection.

Many individuals believe that it is cosmetically more attractive to have a tanned skin and go to a tanning salon where they are exposed to artificial ultraviolet light to maintain a tan all year long. Artificial ultraviolet is just as damaging to the skin as sunlight.

The FDA approved an NDA for ecamsule, which protects the skin against UVA, which penetrates the dermal layer of the skin and causes long-term damage.[32] The use of SPF factors provides consumers with a way to compare sunscreens that protect against UVB, and the FDA is considering establishing a new system for consumers to use when choosing a sunscreen product for protection against UVA. The system would use stars, 1 star for minimal protection and 4 stars for the highest degree of protection.[33]

If the skin is not protected and sunburn occurs, temporary relief can be obtained from OTC products containing external analgesics (hydrocortisone and local anesthetics, as discussed earlier in this chapter), which will reduce irritation and minor pain of the skin. Sunburn that covers an extensive area or a sensitive area of the skin, or results in blistering of the skin, should be treated by a physician.[18]

Products

Most sunscreens have a combination of drugs to provide protection against UVA and UVB. Popular combinations include Aveeno Continuous Protection Sunblock, Bull Frog Quik Gel, Coppertone Sport, PreSun Ultra, Neutrogena Healthy Defense Oil-free Sunblock, and Sea & Ski Advanced Sunscreen.

Monograph sunscreens

Drug category and indications for use

Drugs that are sunscreens are topical dermatological products that protect the skin against sunburn.

Monograph drugs

Several different chemical classifications of drug are monograph sunscreens. Table 8.7 lists the specific FDA approved drugs and includes the type of ultraviolet light protection of each and the mode of action of each.

Mode of action

Sunscreens that are derived from organic chemicals must absorb at least 85% of the ultraviolet light between 290 and 320 nm. These drugs absorb the energy of the light, resulting in a change in the actual chemical composition of the drug and a decrease in the amount of drug available for protection as the

Table 8.7 Categories of FDA approved drugs for sun protection, classified as absorbers or reflectors for specific ranges of ultraviolet (UV) light protection

Drug category	Range of UV protection
Para-aminobenzoic acid derivatives: PABA, padimate O (octyldimethyl PABA), glyceryl aminobenzoate, ethyl-[bis(hydroxypropyl)] aminobenzoate	UVB absorber
Benzophenones derivatives: dioxybenzone, oxybenzone, sulisobenzone	UVB and UVA absorber
Cinnamate derivatives: cinoxate, diethanolamine methoxycinnamate, octinoxate (formerly octyl methoxycinnamate)	UVB absorber
Salicylate derivatives: homosalate, octisalate (formerly octyl salicylate), trolamine salicylate.	UVB absorber
Other organic chemical compounds	
Octocrylene	UVB absorber
Ensulizole	UVB absorber
Avobenzone (Parsol 1789)	UVA-1 absorber
Ecamsule	UVB and UVA-1 absorber
Meradimate	UVA-2 absorber
Inorganic chemical compounds	
Titanium dioxide	UVB, UVA reflecting agent
Zinc oxide	UVB, UVA blocking agent

length of time exposed to the sun increases. These products should be reapplied every 2 to 3 hours.

Titanium dioxide, an inorganic drug, acts by reflecting the ultraviolet light away from the skin, and there is no change in its chemical composition. Zinc oxide, another inorganic drug, acts by physically blocking the ultraviolet light from reaching the skin and is also not affected by the ultraviolet light. Both of these products do not deteriorate with sun exposure and should be reapplied after the individual goes swimming or sweats profusely.[31]

Warnings and precautions

These products are for external use only and individuals should avoid contact with the eyes. If irritation or a skin rash develops, individuals should stop use of the product; if the irritation or rash does not improve, a physician should be consulted.

Recommended use

Suncreens may be applied liberally to the skin of adults and infants over 6 months of age before exposure to sunlight; a physician should be consulted if the infant is less than 6 months old. Sunscreens should be reapplied after swimming or extensive sweating. If the product is labeled as water resistant, it should be reapplied after 40 minutes in the water; if labeled as very water resistant, it is reapplied after 80 minutes.[31]

New drug application sunscreens

Drug category and indications for use
Suncreens prevent epidermal and/or dermal damage from sunlight.

New drug application
Avobenzone and ecamsule.

Mode of action
Avobenzone absorbs UVA-1 rays and ecamsule absorbs UVA-2 rays in sunlight to prevent skin damage.

Warnings and precautions
An individual using a sunscreen should keep the product out of eyes and stop use if irritation or a skin rash develops. If the irritation or rash does not improve, a physician should be consulted.

Recommended use
Sunscreens should be applied to the skin of adults and infants over 6 months of age before exposure to sunlight and reapplied as necessary, especially after swimming or perspiring. Consult a physician for use in infants less than 6 months old.

Products
Avobenzone and ecamsule are combined with octocrylene in Anthelios SX. Avobenzone appears in many other sunscreen products.

Topical antimicrobial drugs

When the integrity of the skin is damaged, the risk of infection is increased. The FDA has approved the use of antiseptics and antibiotics as topical OTC drugs to reduce the risk of infection. If a skin infection does occur, it requires treatment by a physician. Diagnosis of the cause of the infection is beyond the capabilities of untrained individuals, and inappropriate use of antibiotics would increase the risk of creating resistant strains of bacteria.

The first step in proper wound care is cleaning the area with non-irritating skin cleansers, drying the area, application of a topical first aid cream, and protecting the damaged skin by covering it with a sterile bandage. The manufacturer of Band-Aid bandages makes a sterile bandage that contains topical antibiotics in the protective pad, which eliminates the need for applying an antibiotic cream or ointment to minor wounds.

First aid topical antiseptics

Monograph antiseptics

Topical antiseptics are used to clean the skin or minor cuts, scrapes, or burns. Products containing alcohol, isopropyl alcohol, phenol, and iodine tincture will cause pain if applied to broken skin. If the injured skin is to be covered, antiseptics should be removed from the skin by washing or should be thoroughly dried on the skin before a bandage is applied.

Drug category and indications for use

First aid antiseptics are used topically to inhibit microbial growth on the intact skin and reduce the risk of infection in minor cuts, scrapes, and burns.[34]

Monograph ingredients

Alcohol (48 to 95% ethyl alcohol), isopropyl alcohol (50 to 91.3%; 70% isopropyl alcohol is known as rubbing alcohol), hexylresorcinal (0.1%) hydrogen peroxide (3%), iodine tincture, povidone-iodine (5 to 10%), phenol (0.5 to 1.5%), benzalkonium chloride (0.1 to 0.13%), benzethonium chloride (0.1 to 0.2%), and methylbenzethonium chloride (0.13 to 5%).[34]

Mode of action

Antiseptics are drugs that are either microbiostatic or microbiocidal if they remain on the skin for a sufficient amount of time.

Warnings and precautions

General warnings for these drugs include the following:[34] 'this product is for external use only and should not be used around the eyes or mucous membranes, on animal bites, deep or puncture wounds, serious burns, or a large area of the body. If the individual's condition worsens or has not improved within 7 days, a physician should be consulted.'

Specific warnings for specific drugs include the following:[34] (1) alcohol and isopropyl alcohol should not be used near an open flame or fire because they are flammable; (2) phenol containing products should not be bandaged; and (3) iodine containing products should not be used by individuals who are allergic to iodine and they may temporarily stain the skin and clothing.

Recommended use

Antimicrobial drugs should be applied topically to the affected area to clean the skin or minor wound, or they may be applied to the wound after cleaning with water to prevent infection. The area should be allowed to dry before applying a sterile bandage. The product may be applied one to three times a day.

Products

Alcohol, isopropyl alcohol and hydrogen peroxide are available from many generic manufacturers, benzalkonium chloride (Bactine Original First Aid

Liquid with lidocaine, Band-Aid Antiseptic Hurt Free with lidocaine, Neosporin Neo To Go Spray with proxamine), and povidone iodine (Betadine). NOTE: Lidocaine in not recommended for use in children under 2 years of age.

Rx–OTC switched antimicrobial drugs

Drug category and indications for use
Chlorhexidine is a topical antiseptic used to inhibit microbial growth on intact skin or on minor cuts.

New drug application
Chlorhexidine 4% and chlorhexidine with isopropyl alcohol are approved skin wound cleansers and general skin cleansing agents.[35]

Warnings and precautions
Wounds involving more than superficial layers of the skin should not be treated with chlorhexidine. Chlorohexidine should not be used repeatedly as a skin cleanser unless directed by a physician.[35]

Products
Chlorhexidine (Hibiclens Liquid), chlorhexidine and isopropyl alcohol (Hibistat).

First aid topical antibiotics

Drug category and indications for use
An antibiotic drug contains a chemical substance produced by a microorganism that is used topically to inhibit the growth or to kill bacteria on the skin.[36]

Monograph ingredients
Bacitracin 500 Units, neomycin 3.5 mg, and polymyxin B sulfate 10 000 Units are monograph antibiotics.

Mode of action
Bacitracin interferes with amino acids needed for synthesis of bacterial cell walls of Gram-positive bacteria. Neomycin inhibits protein synthesis by binding to the 30S subunit of microbial transfer ribonucleic acid (tRNA), which is found in Gram-negative bacteria and several types of Gram-positive bacteria but not in humans. Polymyxin B is a microcidal surface active agent that alters phospholipids in the cell wall of Gram-negative bacteria.[37]

Warnings and precautions
The individual should not use these products around the eyes, on mucous membranes, or on a large area of the body. If the individual's condition worsens or does not improve in 7 days, a physician should be consulted. If

the individual develops skin irritation or a rash, use of the product should be stopped; if the problem does not improve, a physician should be consulted. Deep puncture wounds, bites, or serious burns require treatment by a physician.

If an individual is allergic to the antibiotic or any ingredient in the product, it should not be used. Neomycin has the greatest risk of causing an allergic response.[36]

Recommended use

Apply a small amount of the product on the skin up to three times a day. A sterile bandage may be applied after application to keep the wound clean.

Products

Bacitracin and neomycin are available from generic manufacturers. Bacitracin is usually combined with neomycin or polymyxin B, or both, because it does not affect Gram-negative bacteria. The monograph does not permit use of polymyxin B as a single ingredient product.

Combination products: Bacitracin and polymyxin B (Polysporin Ointment and Band-Aid Plus Antibiotic Adhesive Bandage), neomycin and polymyxin B (Neosporin Maximum Strength Plus; also contains proxamine, a local anesthetic), bacitracin, neomycin, and polymyxin B (Neosporin First Aid Antibiotic Ointment).

Topical antifungal drugs

Dermatophytes are fungal organisms that depend on keratin, the dead surface layers of the epidermis, for their sustenance. They also infect hair and nails, which are keratin structures. Tinea pedis (athlete's foot), tinea corporis (ringworm), and tinea cruris (jock itch) are the most common fungal infections affecting the epidermis and they are amenable to self-care. Tinea can be spread by direct contact or contact with contaminated surfaces, such as a wet shower room floors, one of the most common sites for spreading tinea pedis. Good personal hygiene practices that keep the skin clean and dry are important in preventing and treating fungal infections.

Conditions favoring the growth of fungi include moisture and heat, which accounts for the sites of the body affected. Symptoms include itching, erythema, flaking, and cracking of the skin. Infections of the scalp and body usually produce a circular pattern, hence the name ringworm. Individuals who are immunosuppressed or taking immunosuppressing drugs are at greater risk of fungal infections than normal individuals. OTC topical hydrocortisone should not be used for treating symptoms of these infections because it will make the problem worse.

Monograph drugs

Drug category and indications for use
Topical antifungal drugs are used to relieve itching, scaling, redness, and burning associated with athlete's foot, jock itch and ringworm.[38]

Monograph ingredients
Clotrimazole (1%), miconazole (2%), tolnaftate (1%), undecylenic acid and its salts (10 to 25%).[38]

Mode of action
Tolnaftate and undecylenic acid and its salts (calcium, copper, and zinc undecylenate) inhibit fungal growth. Miconazole and clotrimazole inhibit synthesis of ergosterol, a component specific to the cell wall of fungi.[37–39]

Warnings and precautions
These products should not be used around the eyes or on mucous membranes.

Recommended use
The individual should apply the product daily on the skin around the toes for up to 4 weeks for athlete's foot. If there is no improvement within 2 weeks, a physician should be consulted. The individual should apply the product daily to the affected area for 2 weeks for jock itch and ringworm. These products should not be used in children under 2 years of age without consulting a physician. These products are not effective for tinea infections on the scalp or nails.[38]

Products
Tolnaftate (Tinactin Foot Powder and Spray and Tinactin Antifungal Jock Itch Powder, Ting Foot and Jock Itch Cream, and Lamisil AF Defense Powder); undecylenic acid (Tineacide Cream, FungiCure Anti-Fungal Liquid).

Rx–OTC switched antifungal drugs

Drug category and indications for use
Topical antifungal drugs are used to relieve itching, scaling, redness, and burning associated with athlete's foot, jock itch, and ringworm.[40]

Active ingredients
Terbinafine and butenafine.

Mode of action
Terbinafine and butenafine inhibit synthesis of ergosterol, a component specific to the fungal cell wall.[37]

Warnings and precautions

Terbinafine 1% and butenafine 1% products have the same warnings. These products should not be used on the nails or scalp and should not be used around the eyes. If the product gets in the individual's eye or eyes, thorough washing with water is necessary. These products are not to be used by women for vaginal yeast infections. If skin irritation occurs, the individual should stop using the products. If the irritation does not improve, the individual should consult a physician.

Recommended use

Terbinafine and butenafine may be applied twice a day for 7 days or once a day for 4 weeks for treatment of athlete's foot. They should be applied to the skin or genital area daily for 2 weeks for treatment of jock itch. These products should not be used by individuals under 12 years of age.[40]

Products

Clotrimazole (Lotrimin AF Anti Jock Itch Powder, Lotrimin AF Anti Fungal Cream), miconazole (Desenex Powder and Spray, Lotrimin AF Spray, Micatin Spray), terbinafine (Lamisil AT Cream, Lamisil AT for Women), butenafine (Lotrimin Ultra AF Antifungal Cream).

Topical antiviral drugs

Warts are caused by human papillomaviruses, which affect the basal layer of skin cells, causing hyperproliferation of epidermal skin cells. Most warts on the skin have a rough, cauliflower appearance and are located predominately on the hands, fingers, feet, knees, and genital areas. There is no OTC treatment for genital warts, or warts on the face or lips.[41]

Warts are contagious and may be spread by direct skin to skin contact, or by skin contact with contaminated inanimate objects. The virus has an incubation period that ranges from 1 to 9 months. Normal shedding of the keratin layer of the epidermis carries the virus with it.

OTC treatment of warts includes the use of keratolytic drugs that remain on the skin for prolonged periods of time. Flexible collodion is the usual pharmaceutical vehicle for keratolytic drug solutions used to treat warts, corns, or calluses. It is a solution of nitrocellulose (pyroxylin) in either ether or acetone, which quickly evaporates after application to the affected area of the skin, leaving a transparent film on the skin.

Keratolytics may also be applied to the skin in the form of a plaster, a pad with a keratolytic drug on a synthetic material that uses adhesive to keep the pad on the skin for a prolonged period of time.

OTC home products that produce a cryotherapeutic type condition are now available for the treatment of warts. Their main advantage is a much shorter treatment time compared with keratolytic therapy. If OTC treatment is unsuccessful, a physician may use liquid nitrogen cryotherapy or some other technique to remove warts.

Monograph drugs (keratolytics)

Drug category and indications for use
Wart removers cause a softening of the keratin in the epidermal layers of the skin to remove common or plantar warts.[41]

Monograph ingredient
Salicylic acid is the only monograph drug. The concentration of salicylic acid varies depending on the formulation used in the product. Products that are plasters contain 12 to 40% salicylic acid and flexible collodion solutions contain 5 to 17%.[41]

Mode of action
A keratolytic drug destroys the integrity of the intracellular matrix of cell walls, causing a softening that increases the shedding of the epidermis. As the keratolytic reaches the basal layer, the virus is also affected and shed with the epidermal cells.

Warnings and precautions
These products should not be used around the eyes or on mucous membranes; broken, irritated, or reddened skin; or the genitals. This product should not be used if the individual has diabetes or poor circulation, and it should not be used on birthmarks, moles (nevi), or warts that have hair growing from them. If the wart becomes very red, sore, or drains fluid, or if numbness or a tingling sensation develops, the product should be stopped and a physician consulted.[41]

Flexible collodion products should not be inhaled and should not be used near an open flame. The bottle should be capped tightly when not in use and not stored near flames or a heated area.

Recommended use
The products are applied only to the wart and not the surrounding skin, after it has been washed, soaked in or with warm water for 5 minutes, and patted dry. Salicylic acid solution may be applied once or twice a day after washing the area. Salicylic acid in plaster formulations may be reapplied in 48 hours after removing the old plaster and cleaning the area. Most warts are removed within 1 to 2 weeks, but the product may be used up to a maximum of 12 weeks.[41]

Products
Salicylic acid: (Compound W, Curad Mediplast, Duo Film Wart Remover, Dr. Scholl's Clear Away Wart Remover, Transversal, Wart Care, Wartner Wart Remover).

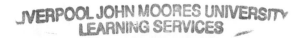

New drug application (cryotherapy)

Drug therapy and indications for use
Cryotherapy uses extreme cold temperature to remove warts.

New drug application
Dimethyl ether packages with butane have received FDA approval as a wart removal system.[42]

Mode of action
Application of extreme cold causes a blister to form under the wart to disrupt and free it from the epidermal layer. The destroyed epidermal tissue sloughs off, removing the virus.

Warnings and precautions
These products are extremely flammable. Do not smoke while applying them and do not use near an open flame; store away from heat. They should be used in a well-ventilated area and inhalation should be avoided. An aerosol product is not sprayed directly on to the skin; it is sprayed on the applicator supplied with the product and then applied to the wart.[43]

Recommended use
Individuals should apply the drug to the skin using applicators that are supplied in the package. Applicators should not be reused. Product may be reapplied but should not be used on the same wart more than four times.[43]

Products
Dimethyl ether (DME) and butane (Compound W Freeze Off, Dr. Scholl's Freeze Away, and Wartner's Plantar Wart Removal System).

Corn and callus removers

Corns and calluses are excessive thickness or growth of the keratinized outer layer of the epidermis. They are usually caused by excessive or continuous pressure on the same area of the skin. They occur most frequently on the feet from improperly fitting footwear or on the palms of the hands or fingers from repetitive pressure. Tissues becomes firm or hardened to protect the lower layers of the epidermis.

Drug category and indications of use
Keratolytics soften and remove the excess keratinized layers of skin.[44]

Monograph drugs
Salicylic acid 12 to 40% is used in a plaster formulation and 12 to 17.6% is used in a flexible collodion solution.[44]

Mode of action
A keratolytic drug destroys the integrity of the intracellular matrix of cell walls, causing a softening that increases the shedding of the epidermis.

Warnings and precautions
The warnings and precautions for salicylic acid used as a corn or callus remover are the same as those described above for wart removal.

Recommended use
The affected area is washed and dried before topical application of the product to the corn or callus. The product may be reapplied in 48 hours for a period up to 14 days. If the condition gets worse or does not improve, a physician or podiatrist should be consulted.[44]

Products
Salicylic acid (Dr. Scholl's Corn Cushions, Dr. Scholl's Maximum Strength Corn Remover, Dr. Scholl's Corn/Callus Remover, Dr. Scholl's Callus pads.)

Ingrown toenail relief

Ingrown toenails are primarily the result of improper trimming or clipping of the nails. Proper grooming should include trimming the nail straight across and not rounding the edges. If the nail is improperly trimmed, the edges of the nail can grow into the skin tissue and may cause pain, inflammation, and swelling. Improperly fitted shoes can also cause this condition through undue pressure on the side of the toe. There is no OTC cure for an ingrown toenail, but the FDA has approved sodium sulfide (1%) to help to relieve pain and discomfort.

Sodium sulfide

Drug category and indications for use
An ingrown toenail relief product relieves pain or discomfort when applied to the toenail.[45]

Monograph ingredient
Sodium sulfide (1%) in a gel vehicle is a monograph drug.

Mode of action
A toenail relief product softens the nail or hardens the nail bed, producing relief from pressure on the tissue around the nail and relieving pain.[45]

Warnings and precautions
This product is for external use only and should not be applied to any open sore or broken skin. Individuals with diabetes, gout, or poor circulation should consult a physician before using this product. This product must be used with the retainer ring provided in the package. If redness or swelling of the toe occurs, if a discharge is present around the nail, or if there is no relief of symptoms within 7 days, the product should be stopped and a physician consulted.[11]

Recommended use

The affected toe is washed and dried before placing the retainer ring on the toe with the open slot over the area where the ingrown toenail and the skin meet. The ring should be smoothed down firmly and the gel applied to the slot in the ring. The round center section of a bandage strip should be applied directly over the gel-filled ring and placed around the toe. This procedure should be performed in the morning and evening for up to 7 days or until the pain and discomfort are relieved. This product should not be used on children under 12 years of age.[45]

Product

Dr. Scholl's Ingrown Toenail Pain Reliever

Acne

Acne is a condition involving the sebaceous glands and hair follicles (pilose-baceous unit), which arise in the dermal layer of the skin and pass through the epidermis to the surface of the skin. Sebum, an oily secretion, remains on the skin, acting as a retardant to moisture loss and providing lubrication of the skin to prevent chapping. Sebum that is not cleansed from the skin may act as an irritant or may block the gland's opening, resulting in blemishes or comedones (pimples) on the skin. Bacteria normally present on the skin, *Propionibacterium acnes,* use the lipids in sebum for nutrition and growth, causing further irritation of the skin and development of papules, pustules, nodules or cysts. Topical antibiotic preparations are available as prescription drugs to control the growth of bacteria.[46]

Acne is rated from grade 1 to grade 4, increasing in severity as the values increase. Mild to moderate acne may respond to OTC products; more severe acne, characterized by pustules and cysts, requires treatment by a physician.

Acne predominately affects adolescents because of the increase in hormone production during this period, especially androgenic compounds. Testosterone and dihydrotestosterone stimulate sebum production. Heat and humidity contribute to the problem, as does the use of oily substances in facial lotions, sunscreens, and cosmetics. Working in kitchens of restaurants, especially fast-food establishments, where the atmosphere is humid and cooking oils are present in the environment exacerbates the problem. The face, upper chest, and back are the areas most commonly affected.

The skin must be cleaned and dried frequently, but harsh soaps and vigorous scrubbing are to be discouraged because the irritation they cause may worsen acne. Numerous acne face-washes or scrubs, and cleansing pads containing salicylic acid or benzoyl peroxide, are available as the initial step in acne treatment. Some products are tinted to mask blemishes, making them less obvious.

Manufacturers of acne products are now marketing a combination of three products as a single system or treatment package for acne. These treatment packages contain a medicated skin wash, which may contain an active drug; a skin toner (a liquid rinse with no active ingredient); and a medicated therapy treatment to be applied after washing and drying the skin.

Rosacea is a dermatological condition inaccurately referred to as adult acne because of its general appearance. It is characterized by vasodilatation of small blood vessels in the skin of the face around the nose, cheeks, chin and forehead, producing redness and skin blemishes. Individuals with rosacea do not have comedones. There is no OTC treatment for this condition.

Drug category and indications for use
Acne products reduce the number of acne blemishes, acne pimples, blackheads (open comedones), and whiteheads (closed comedones).[47]

Monograph ingredients
Salicylic acid (0.5 to 2%), sulfur (3 to 10%) when it is used as a single ingredient in a product, sulfur (3 to 8%) when it is used in a combination product, and resorcinol (2%) or resorcinol monoacetate (3%) when it is combined with sulfur.[47]

Benzoyl peroxide (2.5 to 10%) is not included in the final monograph, but the FDA allows it to continue in OTC products while it evaluates reports of an increase in risk of skin tumors in some animals. The FDA's advisory group did not find evidence that benzoyl peroxide caused skin tumors or caused skin tumors to grow faster in human studies.[48]

Mode of action
Salicylic acid has a keratolytic effect and removes the epidermal layer of the skin, the site of acne blemishes. Sulfur has mild antibacterial and antifungal activity, which may prevent microbial growth. Resorcinol may be combined with sulfur to improve the efficacy of sulfur, but it is not used alone. Benzoyl peroxide has antimicrobial activity through its ability to release oxygen in human tissues.[47,48]

Warnings and precautions
If the individual uses more than one acne medication at the same time, the skin may become excessively dry, causing skin irritation. If this occurs, only one medication should be used. If the individual has discomfort from a combination of products recommended by a physician, the physician should be consulted.

If excessive skin irritation occurs when using a sulfur product, use should be stopped and a physician consulted. Sulfur products containing resorcinol should not be used on broken skin or on a large area of the body.[47]

Benzoyl peroxide may irritate the skin and produce erythema and dryness. It increases the skin's sensitivity to sunlight and individuals are advised to use a sunscreen if they go outdoors. Benzoyl peroxide may cause bleaching and discoloration of clothing.

Recommended use

The individual should clean the skin thoroughly before using any acne product, and apply a thin coating to the affected areas up to three times a day. It is recommended that benzoyl peroxide treatment begins by using it once a day, increasing the number of daily applications if no skin irritation occurs.

Products

Salicylic acid (Biore Blemish Cleanser, Bye Bye Blemish Antiacne Wash, Clean & Clear Continuous Control Acne Wash, Clean & Clear Advantage Acne Cleanser, Clearasil Ultra Daily Face Wash, Clearasil Deep Pore Cleaning Pads, Cuticura Treatment Foaming Face Wash, Neutragena Oil Free Wash, Neutragena Acne Stress Control, Oxy Face Wash, Oxy Face Scrub, Oxy Cleansing Pads, Zapzyt Adult Acne Clearing Gel), salicylic acid and resorcinol (Clearasil Acne Control Adult Cream), benzoyl peroxide (Clean & Clear Persa Gel, Clearsil Ultra, Clearasil Daily Acne Control Vanishing Cream, Neutragena On the Spot Vanishing Formula, Oxy Spot Treatment, Proactiv Renewing Cleanser, Proactiv Repairing Solution, Zapzyt Treatment Bar, Zapzyt Maximum Strength Acne Gel).

Hyperproliferation skin conditions (scaly dermatitis)

Dandruff, seborrhea, and psoriasis are skin conditions in which there is an excessive rate of skin growth or turnover that results in noticeable thickening or shedding of the outer keratinized layer of the skin. These conditions are also referred to as scaly dermatitis. The rate of epidermal turnover in dandruff is approximately twice the normal, in seborrhea it is around five times greater than normal, and in psoriasis it is much greater. Psoriasis has aspects of being an immune disorder, and severe cases require referral to a physician for proper treatment.[49]

Dandruff affects the scalp, the excess epidermal cells appearing as dry, white flakes. The higher levels of a fungus, *Pityrosporum ovale*, on the scalp of individuals with dandruff contribute to the condition because it converts sebum lipids in free fatty acids, which act as skin irritants.

Seborrhea occurs around the scalp, ears, eyebrows, or other areas of the body. The flaking epidermal cells are oily and have a yellow color, and the skin is irritated, itchy, and red. Infant seborrhea is referred to as cradle cap because it occurs on the top of the head of infants. It is only treated by washing the scalp with baby shampoo and generally is a temporary condition that tends to resolve itself as the infant gets a little older.

Psoriasis may occur anywhere on the body, but the wrists, elbows, and knees are the areas that are most frequently affected. The skin appears thick and scaly, with redness and itching. Severe psoriasis appears as white scales or thick plaques and the skin is itchy and inflamed. When the scales break off, the capillaries in the skin and are visible and bleeding can occur. This condition is known as the Auspitz sign.[50]

Shampoos with surface-active agents disperse the epidermal flakes for easy removal when the hair is washed. Shampoos may contain keratoplastic, keratolytic, or cytostatic drugs to treat these conditions.

Dandruff

Drug category and indications
Antidandruff drugs may be used to reduce or eliminate the scaling associated with dandruff.[51]

Monograph drugs
Sulfur (2 to 5%) is a keratoplastic drug; salicylic acid (1.8 to 3%) is a keratolytic drug; and pyrithione zinc (0.95 to 2%), selenium sulfide (1%), micronized selenium sulfide (0.6%), coal tar (0.5 to 5%), and coal tar (1.8%) plus menthol (1.5%) are cytostatic drugs.[51,52]

Mode of action
Keratoplastics (sulfur) and keratolytic drugs (salicylic acid) soften the epidermal skin by affecting the intercellular matrix of cell walls. Keratolytics are more effective and cause the epidermal cells to be sloughed off. Cytostatic drugs inhibit cell turnover but the mechanism is not fully understood.[51]

Warnings and precautions
The products should not be used around the eyes, but if contact occurs, the area should be rinsed thoroughly with water. If the individual's condition does not improve or gets worse after regular use, a physician should be consulted. If the condition affects a large portion of the body, a physician should be consulted. These products should not be used in children under 2 years of age without consulting a physician.[51,52]

Coal tar products sensitize the skin to sunlight and the individual should use a sunscreen before going outdoors. Coal tar products should not be used for prolonged periods of time without consulting a physician. If a cream or ointment formulation is used, it should not be used around the rectum or genital area unless directed by a physician. If an individual uses OTC psoriasis products, the individual should notify the physician if treatment with ultraviolet light is being prescribed.[51]

Recommended use
Products that are used as shampoos should be applied to the scalp and then washed off, and may be used twice a week. Products formulated as lotions, creams, or ointments may be applied to the affected scalp from one to four times a day.

Products
Coal tar (Denorex Dandruff Shampoo and Conditioner Therapeutic), sulfur and salicylic acid (Sebulex Medicated Dandruff Shampoo), salicylic acid (Denorex Shampoo), selenium sulfide (Selsun Blue), zinc pyrithione (AXE Anti-Dandruff Shampoo, Garnier Fructis Hair Care Fortifying 2 in 1 Shampoo, Gillette Anti-Dandruff Shampoo, Head & Shoulders Classic Clean Dandruff Shampoo, Head & Shoulders Dry Scalp Care Shampoo, Head & Shoulders Refresh Dandruff Shampoo, Matrix Men Anti-Dandruff Shampoo, Neutragena T-Gel Dandruff Shampoo, Pert Plus Dandruff Away Shampoo, Suave for Men 2 in 1 Shampoo).

Rx–OTC switch: ketoconazole

Drug category and indications for use
Ketoconazole, an antifungal drug, helps to control flaking, scaling, and itching caused by dandruff.[53]

Rx–OTC switch drug
Ketaconazole 1%.

Mode of action
Ketaconazole has antifungal activity and inhibits the growth of *P. ovale*, which is present on the scalp and contributes to the symptoms associated with dandruff. If a rash appears, the product should be stopped. If the condition gets worse or does not improve within 2 to 4 weeks, the a physician should be consulted.[48,53]

Warnings and precautions
Ketaconazole should not be used on broken or inflamed skin. Contact with the eyes should be avoided; if contact occurs, the eyes should be washed thoroughly with water.[53]

Recommended use
The hair is washed thoroughly with the shampoo and rinsed with water. This is repeated in 3 to 4 days for up to 8 weeks. The product should not be used on children under 12 years of age.[53]

Product
Ketaconazole (Nizoral A-D Shampoo).

Seborrhea

Drug category and indications for use
Antiseborrhea products help to control and relieve the irritation and itching of seborrheic dermatitis.[51]

Monograph ingredients
Keratoplastics (sulfur), keratolytics (salicylic acid), and cytostatic drugs (pyrithione zinc, selenium sulfide, and coal tar).

Mode of action

Keratoplastics and keratolytics soften epidermal skin, allowing cells to slough off easily when the hair and skin are washed. Cytostatic drugs inhibit cell turnover to prevent build-up of excess keratinized epithelial cells.

Warnings and precautions

Contact with the eyes should be avoided. If the condition affects a large area of the body, a physician should be consulted before using any of these products. If the condition does not improve or if it gets worse, a physician should be consulted. These products are not recommended for use in children under 2 years of age.

Infant seborrhea (cradle cap) should not be treated with these products; a shampoo formulated for babies should be used. If baby shampoo does not improve infant seborrhea, the caregiver should consult a physician.

Products

Salicylic acid (Denerox Shampoo), zinc pyrithione (SkinZinc Spray for Seborrhea; the product label for this drug recommends that it be used in individuals 18 years of age or older), coal tar (Neutragena T-Gel).

Psoriasis

Drug category and indications for use

Drugs for treating psoriasis relieve the itching, flaking, and inflammation associated with psoriasis.[51,52]

Monograph ingredients

Only coal tar and salicylic acid are monograph drugs for treating the symptoms associated with psoriasis.[50–52]

Mode of action

Coal tar and salicylic acid act in the manner described for dandruff.

Warnings and precautions

If psoriasis affects a large area of the body, a physician should be consulted before using these products. Contact with the eyes should be avoided. If the condition does not improve or gets worse, the individual should contact a physician.

Coal tar products sensitize the skin to sunlight and the individual should use a sunscreen before going outdoors. Coal tar products should not be used for prolonged periods of time without consulting a physician. If a cream or ointment formulation is used, it should not be used around the rectum or genital area unless directed by a physician. If an individual uses OTC psoriasis products, the individual should notify the physician if treatment with ultra-violet light is being prescribed.[51] Product labels for psoriasis products containing coal tar recommend that they be used by individuals 18 years of age or older.

Products

Coal tar (Psoriasin has several formulations, including Psoriasin MultiSymptom Psoriasis Relief Ointment, Liquid, Scalp Liquid, and Gel), salicylic acid (Dermarest Psoriasis Medicated Moisturizer and Dermarest Psoriasis Shampoo, SkinZinc Cream for Psoriasis (this product is recommended for individuals 18 years of age or older)).

Case study exercises

Case 1 KM, a 78-year-old man, tells the pharmacist that the skin on his arms is dry, flaking, and itching. He used hydrocortisone lotion for itching when he had a case of poison ivy and wanted to know if he should buy some for this problem.

The pharmacist asked if he used any moisturizing cream on his arms. KM replied that he never used any skin lotions. The pharmacist suggested that the KM's problem could be caused by dry skin (xerosis), explaining that without any other cause, this was most likely his problem. KM is at risk for dry skin based on his age. Although hydrocortisone will relieve itching, it has no benefit for dry, flaky skin.

The pharmacist recommended that he try using a product like Eucerin or Aveeno twice a day for several days and avoids using ordinary soaps for bathing, trying Cetaphil, a nonsoap skin cleansing agent. He also recommended that warm water rather than hot water be used for bathing. If these suggestions do not relieve KM's symptoms, the pharmacist recommended that he call his doctor.

Case 2 JR, a 17-year-old man, was helping a neighbor to clear some brush from the yard yesterday. He wore gloves but took his shirt off because it was a very hot day. Now he has a rash on his arms and chest that is red, very itchy, and has small skin blisters filled with fluid. The neighbor said there was poison ivy in the yard.

The pharmacist suggests that JR call his doctor because the area of skin exposed to the poison ivy is relatively large and OTC products may not be the most effective manner to treat this problem. However, if JR wanted to try an OTC product, he should use an antipruritic lotion or spray that contained either hydrocortisone, like Cortaid, or a local anesthetic, like Gold Bond Medicated Itch Relief.

Case 3 A 56-year-old woman asks the pharmacist to recommend a product because she has arthritis in her right knee that has been painful for the last 5 days. She has been taking Tylenol to relieve the pain and it provides some relief but her knee pain still limits her activities. Her sister told her to buy capsaisin cream and she wants to know if this is appropriate.

The pharmacist explains that capsaisin is used to relief pain associated with arthritis but that it does not produce its maximum effect for approximately 7 to 10 days. The pharmacist suggests a topical cream that contains external analgesic such as BenGay Cream (camphor, menthol, and methyl salicylate) or Salonpas Arthritis Patch (menthol and methyl salicylate) for more immediate relief.

Case 4 A mother asks the pharmacist if Off Skintastic could be used on her 4-year-old child. She lives in the neighborhood where there are deer and she afraid the child will be bitten by a deer tick.

The pharmacist tells the woman that Skintastic has a high concentration of DEET, an insect repellent that is not recommended for use in young children. He suggests that she use picaridin, an insect repellent that is as effective as DEET for ticks but does not have the same dangerous adverse effects as DEET. The pharmacist also reminds the mother that once the child comes indoors, the insect repellent should be washed off, regardless of the product that is used.

Case 5 A mother asks the pharmacist to recommend a product because her child has head lice.

The pharmacist recommends the mother use Nix or RID lice shampoos. Both must remain on the hair for 10 minutes and should be thoroughly washed from the hair. The hair should be patted dry and a fine-toothed comb should be used to remove nits (larvae) from the base of the hair follicle. The hair should be checked and the process repeated in 7 days if all the lice have not been killed or removed. If the lice remain after the second treatment, the mother should consult the child's doctor because the lice may be resistant to this topical therapy. There are prescription medications that are effective for resistant strains of lice. All other members of the family should be checked to see if they are infected with head lice and should be treated in the same manner if infested.

The mother must be reminded to wash all contaminated clothing in hot water, placing them in the dryer on the hot cycle for 20 minutes. Items that cannot be washed may be sprayed with a pediculicide spray, or they could be stored in a closed, plastic bag for 2 weeks to be certain that both adult lice and the larvae have died.

Case 6 GB cut his hand 3 days ago while working. It is getting swollen and red. He asks the pharmacist for an antibiotic ointment.

The pharmacist tells GB that he must see a physician because the symptoms he describes indicates that the wound could be infected. None of the antibiotic ointments available OTC are for treating an infection. They are only to be used on minor wounds to prevent infections.

Case 7 YT asks the pharmacist what to do about several warts on her hands because they are embarrassing to her. She tried Compound W but the warts came back.

The pharmacist suggests she try home cryotherapy for the warts, a procedure that should destroy the tissue that virus has infected. If this procedure does not rid her of the warts, she should a consult a physician for a more effective treatment.

Case 8 NS is 16 years old and works as a cook in a fast-food restaurant. He asks the pharmacist to recommend a product for his acne. NS has only a few pustules and comedones on his face.

The pharmacist recommends that he should be sure to keep the skin on his face clean and apply an acne product every morning and evening. The pharmacist suggests using a medicated pad to wipe his face during working hours to reduce the amount of oil on the skin surface. NS could use Clear & Clean Persa Gel morning and evening, but he must use a sunscreen if he will be exposed to the sun because the benzoyl peroxide will increase his sensitivity to the sun. He could use Clearsil pads for cleaning his skin at work.

Case 9 CK, a 77-year-old man, complains that his dandruff is getting very bad. He complains that his scalp along his hairline is itching, red, and feels oily. When he combs his hair, there are yellow-looking flakes.

The pharmacist asks CK if he has talked to his doctor about the problem, but CK says he didn't and doesn't like going to see the doctor. The pharmacist suggests that CK may have seborrhea and he should try a medicated shampoo with salicylic acid, such as Denorex Shampoo, twice a week for several weeks to see if it helps his symptoms. If CK doesn't experience any relief, he could try a coal tar shampoo or call his doctor.

References

1. *Decoding the Cosmetic Label.* www.cfsan.fda.gov/~dms/cos-labl.html (accessed March 19, 2009).

2. Marks Jr., JG, Miller JJ, *Lookingbill & Marks' Principles of Dermatology*, 4th edn. Philadelphia, PA: Saunders Elsevier, 2006.
3. Robert WE. Dermatologic problems of older women. *Dermatol Clin* 2006; 24: 271–280.
4. Skin protectant drug products for over-the-counter human use; final monograph. *Fed Regist* 2003; 68: 33362–33381.
5. Wasserbauer N, Ballow M. Atopic dermatitis. *Am J Med* 2009; 122: 121–125.
6. *Hydrocortisone; History of Rule Making*. www.fda.gov/ohms/dockets/ac/05/slides/2005-4099S1_02_FDA-Koenig.ppt (accessed March 18, 2009).
7. External analgesic drug products for over-the-counter human use; amendment of tentative final monograph; notice of proposed rulemaking. *Fed Regist* 1990; 55: 6931–6951.
8. Skin protectant drug products for over-the-counter human use; diaper rash products; proposed rule. *Fed Regist* 1990; 55: 25204–25232.
9. *Poison Ivy*. www.mayoclinic.com/health/poison-ivy/DS00774 (accessed March 18, 2009).
10. *Technu Information*. www.teclabsinc.com/products.cfm?id=1F5604C8-9D05-4675-56129F6D83DF2417&section=1 (accessed March 22, 2009).
11. Marks JG et al. Prevention of poison ivy and poison oak allergic contact dermatitis by quaternium-18 bentonite. *J Am Acad Dermatol* 1995; 33: 212–216.
12. *Ivy Block information*. www.ivyblock.com (accessed March 18, 2009).
13. Skin protectant and external analgesic drug products for over-the-counter human use; proposed rulemaking for poison ivy, poison oak, poison sumac, and insect bites drug products. *Fed Regist* 1989; 54: 40808–40827.
14. Labeling of diphenhydramine containing drug products for over-the-counter human use; final rule. *Fed Regist* 2002; 67: 72555–72559.
15. *Active Ingredients Found in Insect Repellents*. Last updates September 8, 2008. www.eps.gov/pesticides/hea;th/mosquitoes/ai_insectrp.htm. (accessed March 22, 2009).
16. *Updated Information Regarding Insect Repellents*. www.cdc.gov/ncidod/dvbid/westnile/RepellentUpdates.htm (accessed March 22, 2009).
17. *Follow Safety Precautions When Using DEET on Children*. www.aap.org/family/wnv-jun03.htm (accessed March 22, 2009).
18. External analgesic drug products for over-the-counter human use; establishment of a monograph and notice of proposed rulemaking. *Fed Regist* 1979; 44: 69768–69866.
19. Pediculicide drug products for over-the-counter human use; final monograph. *Fed Regist* 1993; 58: 65452–65456.
20. Pediculicide drug products for over-the-counter human use; amendment of final monograph. *Fed Regist* 2003; 68: 75414–75418.
21. *Nix Information*. www.NixLice.com (accessed March 26, 2009).
22. *LiceMD Information*. www.LiceMD.com (accessed March 26, 2009).
23. *Licefreee! Information*. www.licefree.com (accessed March 23, 2009).
24. Stitik TP et al. Pharmacotherapy of arthritis. *Am J Phy Med Rehabil* 2006; 85: (11 Suppl) S15–S28.
25. *Hemorrhoids*. www.webmd.com/a-to-z-guides/hemorrhoids-topic-overview (accessed April 4, 2009).
26. Anorectal drug products for over-the counter human use; establishment of a monograph. *Fed Regist* 1980; 45: 35576–35677.
27. Anorectal drug products for over-the–counter human use; final monograph; final rule. *Fed Regist* 1990; 55: 31776–31783.
28. Antiperspirant drug products for over-the-counter human use; final monograph. *Fed Regist* 2003; 68: 34273–34293.
29. Mirick DK et al. Antiperspirant use and risk of breast cancer. *J Natl Cancer Inst* 2002; 94: 1578–1580.
30. Namer M et al. [The use of deodorants/antiperspirants does not constitute a risk factor for breast cancer.] [Article in French; Abstract in English]. *Bull Cancer* 2008; 95: 871–880.
31. Sunscreen drug products for over-the-counter human use; tentative final monograph. *Fed Regist* 1993; 58: 28194–28302.
32. FDA Approves A New Over-the-counter Sunscreen Product. www.fda.gov/bbs/topics/NEWS/2006/NEW01417.html (accessed February 12, 2009).

33. FDA Proposes New Rule for Sunscreen Products. www.fda.gov/bbs/topics/NEWS/2007?NEW01687.html (accessed March 27, 2009).

34. Topical antimicrobial drug products for over-the–counter human use; tentative final monograph for first aid antiseptic drug products; proposed rule *Fed Regist* 1991; 56: 33644–33680.

35. Hibiclens. www.hibiclens.com/hibi_info.html (accessed April 2, 2009).

36. Topical antimicrobial drug products for over-the-counter human use; final monograph for OTC first aid antibiotic drug products; final rule. *Fed Regist* 1987; 52: 47312–47324.

37. Feldman SR *et al. Handbook of Dermatologic Drug Therapy*. London: Taylor & Francis, 2005.

38. Topical antifungal drug products for over-the-counter human use; final monograph. *Fed Regist* 1993; 58: 49890–49899.

39. Topical antifungal drug products for over-the-counter human use; amendment of final monograph. *Fed Regist* 2002; 67: 5942–5943.

40. *Comparison of Labeling for All Topical Antifungals Treating Athlete's Foot.* http://fda.gov/ohrms/dockets/ac/04/briefing/4036B1_08_Product%20Labeling.htm (accessed April 3, 2009).

41. Wart remover drug products for over-the-counter human use; final monograph. *Fed Regist* 1990; 55: 33246–33256.

42. Wartner Wart Removal System for OTC Use. www.fda.gov/cdrh/pdf3/k032271.pdf (accessed April 4, 2009).

43. *Wartner Information.* http://wartner-us.com/instructions1.htm (accessed April 4, 2009).

44. Corn and callus remover drug products for over-the-counter human use; final monograph; final rule. *Fed Regist* 1990; 55: 33258–33262.

45. Ingrown toenail relief drug products for over-the-counter human use; final rule. *Fed Regist* 2003; 68: 24347–24349.

46. Clarke SB *et al.* Pharmacologic modulation of sebaceous gland activity: mechanisms and clinical applications. *Dermatol Clin* 2007; 25: 137–146.

47. Topical acne products for over-the-counter human use; final monograph; final rule. *Fed Regist* 1991; 56: 41008–41020.

48. Topical drug products containing benzoyl peroxide; required labeling. *Fed Regist* 1995; 60: 9554–9558.

49. Pray WS. *Nonprescription Product Therapeutics*, 2nd edn. Philadelphia, PA: Lippincott Williams & Wilkins, 2006.

50. Menter A *et al.* Guidelines for care and management of psoriasis and psoriatic arthritis. Section 3. Guidelines of care for the management and treatment of psoriasis with topical therapies. *J Am Acad Dermatol* 2009; 60: 643–659.

51. Dandruff, seborrhea dermatitis, and psoriasis drug products for human over-the-counter use; final rule. *Fed Regist* 1991; 56: 63554–63569.

52. Dandruff, seborrhea dermatitis, and psoriasis drug products containing coal tar and menthol for over-the-counter human use; amendment to the monograph. *Fed Regist* 2007; 72: 9849–9852.

53. *Nizoral A-D Ketoconazole Shampoo.* www.nizoral.com/vcrc/drugfacts/listproducts.jhtml (accessed April 4, 2009).

9

Miscellaneous products

Weight loss products

Orlistat

Obesity is a major health concern not only in the USA but worldwide because it is a major risk factor for heart disease and diabetes mellitus. Many untested and ineffective products are widely promoted. The FDA banned ephedra, a drug that stimulates the sympathetic nervous system to suppress appetite centers in the brain, from the marketplace in 2004 because of its serious adverse effects, which included many deaths.[1] Unfortunately, ephedra still appears in many weight-loss supplement products that may be obtained from sources outside the USA via internet purchases.

Bitter orange (*Citrus aurantium*) contains synephrine, a sympathomimetic drug that produces many of the same effects as ephedra and is in many dietary supplements still promoted for weight loss. There is little evidence of its effectiveness as a weight-loss product and it has the same risks of ephedra. It may cause nervousness, irritability, and insomnia and it increases heart rate and blood pressure, increasing the risk of heart attacks and stroke.[2]

Healthy eating habits and physical activity are the most reliable methods that produce weight loss. Many different diets are available, such as low carbohydrates or high protein, but the most significant weight loss occurs when total caloric intake is reduced. Mild exercise increases the expenditure of calories and if used with reduced calorie intake provides the more reliable method for losing weight.

The FDA approved the switch of the prescription drug orlistat to OTC status, and it is the only OTC drug available at this time for weight loss.

Drug category and indications for use
Orlistat will increase weight loss by as much as 25% when combined with a healthy eating plan.[3]

Mode of action

Orlistat inhibits the action of lipases in the stomach and small intestines; these enzymes metabolize dietary fats to forms that can be absorbed, hence orlistat prevents fat absorption and reduces caloric intake.

Warnings and precautions

Transplant recipients should not use orlistat because it interferes with the action of drugs used to prevent organ rejection, particularly cyclosporine. Individuals who have gall bladder problems, kidney stones, pancreatitis, problems with absorbing foods, or who take other weight-loss medications should not use orilstat. Individuals who are not overweight should not take this drug.[3]

Individuals taking warfarin, a blood thinner, or medicines for thyroid disease or diabetes should consult a physician or pharmacist before taking orlistat.[3]

When taking orlistat, a multiple vitamin product containing vitamins A, D, E, K, and beta-carotene should be used daily at bedtime. These vitamins are fat-soluble vitamins and the use of orilstat will affect their absorption from foods.

A well-balanced reduced calorie diet should be eaten while taking orlistat because it produces its effect in the GI tract to prevent fat absorption. Individuals may experience bowel changes, gas, oil spotting, loose stools, and more frequent stools, which may be hard to control. Eating a low-fat diet will reduce these effects.

Recommended dose

Adults and adolescents over 18 years of age should take one capsule with each meal containing fat but not more than three capsules a day.[3] Orlistat is not recommended for individuals under 18 years of age.

Product

The starter package for Alli contains the following: an eating guide and discussion of healthy food choices for a weight-reducing diet; a calorie and fat chart to assist the individual make better choices; and a daily journal that assists the individual in keeping a record of their caloric intake.

Smoking cessation products

The use of tobacco products places a large burden on the healthcare system because of all the deleterious effects it has on the human body. These effects include increasing the risk of heart disease and stroke, bronchitis, chronic obstructive pulmonary disease, emphysema, increased risk of infections such as pneumonia, reduced fertility in women, increased risk to the fetus during the pregnancy and low birthweight infants, and increased cancer risk of the oral cavity, esophagus, stomach, pancreas, lung, and bladder.

Tobacco use is a learned behavior and, like weight control, changing behavior is very difficult for many people. Nicotine is an addictive drug and its effects in the central nervous system are similar to those of other addictive drugs. Nicotine's effects on dopamine receptors is primarily responsible for its pleasurable effects, but it also acts at other neurotransmitter sites to cause arousal, appetite suppression, and suppression of anxiety. The most successful programs to stop smoking have several components. The most important component is the decision on the part of the individual to stop smoking. Once the individual makes this decision and chooses a stop date, the individual must decide the method to employ to insure success.[4,5]

The 'cold turkey' method may work for some people, but unpleasant withdrawal symptoms occur when nicotine use is abruptly stopped, leading many individuals to resume their tobacco habit. Withdrawal symptoms include irritability, anxiety, difficulty in concentration, depression, insomnia, weight gain, and a craving or increased desire to smoke.

The use of nicotine replacement alleviates many of these symptoms, helping the individual to continue with the program to stop smoking. If the individual works with a counselor in a one-on-one situation or with a group of individuals who have the same goal, the chance of succeeding is greatly improved. There are programs where a counselor or health coach is available by toll free phone anytime the individual feels that he or she needs encouragement or help to overcome the desire to resume smoking.

The US Public Health Service published a reference guide of strategies for smoking cessation programs. The guidelines recommend the '5 A's' approach.[6] Healthcare providers should ask, advise, assess, assist, and arrange a program for the individual who decides to quit smoking.

OTC nicotine replacement products are available in several dosage forms: gum, lozenge, and transdermal patches. Each type of product has different rates of onset of action and duration of action, and individuals choose the product type that most appeals to them. Many individuals may have made previous attempts to stop smoking and been unsuccessful with OTC products. The individual should always be encouraged to try again. If OTC product use is not successful, the individual should consult a physician because there are several prescription drugs available that may be appropriate for them to try.

Nicotine replacement products

Drug category and indications for use
OTC nicotine products act on sites in the central nervous system to relieve symptoms of nicotine withdrawal when tobacco use is stopped.[4,5]

Rx–OTC drug
Nicotine

Mode of action

When tobacco use is stopped, the levels of nicotine present in the nervous system decline and this produces withdrawal symptoms that are physically unpleasant. Nicotine replacement products are used in decreasing doses over a period of time to wean the person away from smoking on a precise schedule to minimize symptoms. When the planned doses are stopped, the individual should not experience any unpleasant effects and will stop smoking. Unfortunately, the craving feeling for tobacco that an individual has remains to some degree in most individuals.

Warnings and precautions

No nicotine replacement product may be sold to persons under the age of 18 years of age, and proof of age is required. Prescriptions are required if individuals are under 17 years of age. These products should not be used if a woman is pregnant or breast feeding because they may cause an increased heart rate in the child. Individuals should not continue to smoke if these products are being used. Individuals who have heart disease, a recent heart attack, high blood pressure, or irregular heart rhythms should consult a physician before using these products.

Any individual who experiences a rapid heart rate, nausea, vomiting or dizziness should stop using the product and a physician should be consulted. Individuals should stop using this product when the schedule for tapering doses has reached its scheduled conclusion.

Products that are gums slowly release nicotine from a polacrilex, flavored formulation, and should not be used in individuals who have problems chewing or temporomandibular joint problems. An individual who has dentures, braces, or other dental appliances could consult with the dentist before using a gum. Irritation of oral mucous membrane, hiccups, or gastric upset can occur from use of the gum. Do not eat or drink for 15 minutes before or while using the gum.

Products that are lozenges should not be chewed or swallowed. Individuals may experience nausea, hiccups, or heartburn while using lozenges. Do not eat or drink for 15 minutes before or while using the lozenge.

Products that are transdermal patches should be placed on clean, dry, hair-free, intact skin on the upper body or the upper outside portion of the arm. Patches should be rotated on different parts of the body to reduced possible skin irritation, which could be caused either by the drug or by the adhesive on the patch. A new patch should be used every 24 hours. If vivid dreams occur, remove the patch at bedtime and apply new patch in the morning. The patches may not be cut into separate pieces. All used patches should be disposed of safely.

Recommended dose

When the gum is used, it should be chewed slowly until the individual feels a tingling or flavor sensation. The gum is then placed between the cheek and gum until the sensation subsides, and then the gum is again slowly chewed

Table 9.1 Weekly schedules for doses of Nicorette gum and Committ lozenges		
Weeks	**Nicorette gum[a]**	**Committ lozenge[b]**
1 through 6	1 piece every 1–2 h	1 lozenge every 1–2 h
7 through 9	1 piece every 2–4 h	1 lozenge every 2–4 h
10 through 12	1 piece every 4–8 h	1 lozenge every 4–8 h
Maximum 24 h dose	24 pieces	20 lozenges

[a] If 25 or more cigarettes are smoked per day, use the 4 mg dose; if less than 25 cigarettes per day, use 2 mg dose.
[b] If the first cigarette is smoked within 30 min of waking up after sleeping, use the 4 mg lozenge; if 30 min or more elapse, use the 2 mg dose.

again and the process is repeated. This is known as the 'chew and park' technique. The gum should be 'parked' in different areas to avoid irritation of the oral tissue. The nicotine is absorbed during this time. It should take approximately 30 minutes until the full dose of nicotine is released. If the gum is continually chewed without these periods for absorption, the nicotine is swallowed and is not absorbed from the stomach because of its acid environment. Therefore, the product will not be effective.

The gum is available in 2 and 4 mg doses. The starting dose depends on the number of cigarettes smoked per day. Table 9.1 provides the number of pieces of gum to be used, and the schedule for use.

When the lozenge is used, it should be allowed to fully dissolve in the mouth and it should be moved to different areas to prevent irritation of the oral tissue. The lozenge is available in 2 mg and 4 mg strengths and the strength and number of lozenges to be used is determined by in the amount of time that elapses before the individual smokes the first cigarette of the day after awakening from sleep. See table 9.1 for dose schedule.

When a transdermal patch is used, nicotine is absorbed through the skin at a slower rate than the gum or lozenge, and is released over a longer period of time. It does not act quickly to satisfy the immediate need that an individual may desire. Patches are available in varying strengths: 7 mg, 14 mg, and 21 mg. Starting dosage depends on the number of cigarettes smoke per day. Table 9.2 provides the schedule for use of the patch formulations.

Table 9.2 Recommended dose schedule for Nicoderm CQ and Habitrol Transdermal patches		
	Smoke ≥ 10 cigarettes per day	**Smoke < 10 cigarettes per day**
Step 1 (21 mg patch)	1 patch daily, weeks 1–6	Do not use
Step 2 (14 mg patch)	1 patch daily, weeks 7–8	1 patch daily, weeks 1–6
Step 3 (7 mg patch)	1 patch daily, weeks 9–10	1 patch daily, weeks 7–8

Products

Nicotine gum (Nicorette and generic formulations), nicotine lozenges (Committ), nicotine patches (Nicoderm, Habitrol and generic formulations).

Osteoarthritis (arthritis)

Osteoarthritis (arthritis) is a chronic, progressive disease that primarily affects the aging population. It is often considered to be a phenomenon resulting from 'wearing out' of the body's bone and cartilage structures, but many factors are involved in the disease, including genetic factors, inflammation, obesity, previous injury, and metabolic or endrocrine disorders. Joints in the knees, hips, and hands are most commonly affected.

Articular cartilage in joints allows for smooth pain-free movement and absorbs and distributes pressures resulting primarily from the weight of the body. As cartilage becomes thinner, it is no longer able to function properly, and the joint's synovial fluid becomes less viscous and elastic. The joint space decreases and eventually movement becomes stiff and painful.[7]

Physical therapy with nonweight-bearing exercises helps to relieve stiffness in some individuals. Pharmacotherapy for arthritis involves the use of OTC drugs, acetaminophen, and the nonsteroidal anti-inflammatory drugs (NSAIDs) (see Chapter 5), and prescription NSAIDs. Intra-articular injection of corticosteroids, which have anti-inflammatory properties, provides relief that lasts for a limited time. Injection of hyaluronic acid, a normal constituent of synovial fluid, may restore some normal function for a limited period of time, providing some pain relief.[7]

Glucosamine and glucosamine with chrondroitin are dietary supplements that have demonstrated pain relief without the adverse effects associated with the OTC or prescription drugs. Maximum benefit with glucosamine requires several weeks of continuous use. Current studies have not provided evidence that glucosamine or its combined use with chondroitin have any significant effect on cartilage loss when compared with placebo.[8]

Dietary supplements

Glucosamine

Drug category and indications for use

Glucosamine is an aminoglycan protein used to maintain cartilage.

Mode of action

Glucosamine stimulates synthesis of mucopolysaccharides, components of articular cartilage and synovial fluid. Supplements of glucosamine hydrochloride or glucosamine sulfate may help to restore damaged cartilage and/or may prevent further degradation of cartilage.[9,10]

Warnings and precautions
Glucosamine that is prepared from the exoskeletons of shellfish such as shrimp and crab may precipitate an allergic reaction and should be avoided. It may cause nausea, vomiting, and heartburn.[9,10]

Recommended dose
Glucosamine is recommended in daily doses of 500 to 1500 mg for adults and individuals over the age of 18. The dose may be given as a single dose or it may be divided into two or three doses per day.

Products
Glucosamine hydrochloride or glucosamine sulfate (available from many generic manufacturers).

Chrondroitin sulfate

Drug category and indications for use
Chrondroitin is an aminoglycan that is used to maintain cartilage.

Mode of action
Chrondroitin stimulates synthesis of mucopolysaccharides, components of articular cartilage and synovial fluid. Supplements of chrondition sulfate or chrondroitin combined may help to restore damaged cartilage and/or may prevent further degradation of cartilage.

Warnings and precautions
Chrondroitin may cause gastric irritation and nausea.

Recommended dose
Chrondroitin sulfate may be used in adults or individuals over the age of 18 in doses of 200 mg to 400 mg two or three times a day.

Products
Chrondroitin sulfate (available from many generic manufacturers).
    NOTE: Glucosamine (500 mg) and chrondroitin (400 mg) are frequently used together (Cosamin DS and Osteo BiFlex). There is no evidence that the combination is superior to using glucosamine alone.[8,9]

Hair loss (alopecia)

Hair is protein keratin and may be vellous hair, soft, fine usually unpigmented, or terminal hair, thicker and pigmented. Terminal hair has three stages of growth: anagen (approximately 2 to 6 years), catagen (2 to 3 weeks), and telogen (approximately 12 weeks), a resting stage. As telogen hair is lost, a new cycle of hair growth begins. The anagen stage becomes shorter with each new cycle of growth.[11]

Normal hair is shed at a rate from 50 to 100 hairs a day because telogen hair becomes more loosely connected to the hair follicle. Hair growth and hair loss (alopecia) are affected by many factors including genetic predisposition, nutrition, age, stress, gender, diseases, and drug therapy. Androgenic hormones have the greatest influence on hair growth and loss. Androstenedione and dihydroepiandrosterone from the adrenal gland in men and women, and testosterone and 5-alpha-dihydrotestosterone in men are the principal circulating human androgens. 5-Alpha-dihydrotestosterone is the most potent androgen in the skin and is the major factor that causes androgenic alopecia, male pattern baldness.

Male pattern baldness begins on the crown of the head and extends over a greater portion of the scalp, and in some individuals covers the entire scalp. Terminal hair begins to lose its thickness and becomes finer and is then shed. It is replaced by thinner, vellous hair, which is colorless and much shorter. Male pattern baldness also occurs in women but with a much lower incidence. Women usually lose hair from all areas of the scalp, not just the crown of the head. Male pattern baldness is the only type of alopecia amenable to treatment with OTC drugs.

Minoxidil

Drug category and indications for use
Topical minoxidil is used to regrow hair on the scalp.

Rx–OTC switch drug ingredients
Minoxidil 2% and 5%.

Mode of action
The exact mode of action is unknown but several actions could contribute to hair growth, opeing of potassium channels, through inhibition of normal calcium entry into cells, and possibly increasing the blood supply through its vasodilating action. However, other drugs that cause vasodilatation of the blood vessels in the scalp have not increased hair growth.[11]

Warnings and precautions
Minoxidil carries the following warnings.[12] 'If hair loss is greater than the amount shown on the side of this product's label or if hair loss is on the front of the scalp, the product should not be used because it will not be effective. If the individual has no family history of hair loss, or if hair loss is sudden and patchy, or if it occurs for an unknown reason, minioxidil should not be used. It should not be used on any part of the body except the scalp. Do not use if the scalp is inflamed, irritated, infected, or if any other medication are being used on the scalp. Individual's who have heart disease should not use minoxidil without consulting a phyician. Contact with the eyes should be avoided.'

If an individual experiences chest pain, rapid heart rate, faintness, dizziness, sudden unexplained weight gain, swelling of the hands or feet or if redness and irritation of the scalp occurs, use of the product should be stopped and a physician consulted.

Recommended use
Minoxidil 2% topical solution may be applied to the affected area of the scalp twice a day. Results may not be noticeable for 2 to 4 months, and hair texture and color may change. This product will not produce the same amount of hair growth for all individuals. Continued use is required for continued hair growth. This product is not for use by individuals under 18 years of age.[12,13]

Minoxidil 5% is for use by men only and should not be used by women. Men should stop use and a physician should be consulted if hair growth does not occur in 12 months. Women using 2% minoxidil should stop use and a physician should be consulted if hair growth does not occur in 8 months.[12,13]

Products
Minoxidil (Women's Rogaine 2% Solution, Men's Rogaine 5% Solution and 5% foam).

Adaptogen

An adaptogen is considered to be a nontoxic substance that allows the body to respond to a variety of stresses, including emotional and physical factors. Most adaptogens have a long history of use in Chinese medicine. The best known and most frequently studied is ginseng. *Panax ginseng*, also known as Asian ginseng, Chinese ginseng, or Korean red ginseng, has been promoted for a great number of conditions. There is evidence that it may have a positive effect on cholesterol metabolism through its antioxidant actions. It may improve the immune system's response in some respiratory conditions, and it may reduce blood glucose levels in individuals who have type 2 diabetes.[14]

American ginseng, *Panax quinquefolius*, is an alternative to Chinese ginseng and contains the same ginsenosides that are considered to be the active constituents in the plant. Siberian or Russian ginseng is *Eleutherococcus senticosus*, a less-expensive alternative that does not contain ginsenosides.[14,15]

In addition to ginseng products available as dietary supplements, many consumer beverages and multivitamin products are marketed that contain ginseng, including bottled water and energy or sports drinks. These products are promoted to improve an individual's immunity and to increase a feeling of well-being and stamina.

Ginseng

Drug category and indications for use
Ginseng is a dietary supplement that may improve lipid metabolism, blood glucose levels, and immunity, increase energy and stamina, improve memory, reduce GI problems, reduce inflammation, improve a cancer patient's general health, and improve heart disease.[14]

Mode of action
The mechanism of action for the various effects of these ginsenosides remains unclear.

Warnings and precautions
Individuals who have allergic reactions to any *Panax* species should not use ginseng. Ginseng may reduce the effectiveness of warfarin in individuals requiring anticoagulation therapy. Individuals who have type 2 diabetes should consult their physician before using ginseng.[14]

Recommended dose
Adults doses of 100 to 200 mg of ginseng extract (4% ginsenosides) may be taken once or twice a day for 12 weeks. Ginseng is not recommended for use in individuals under 18 years of age.[14]

Products
Ginsana and many generic forms of ginseng are available.

Memory loss and dementia

Ginkgo biloba

Ginkgo biloba extracts are dietary supplements that have been promoted as memory enhancers for many years. Forgetfulness is associated frequently with normal aging, and more severe memory loss and dementia are associated with a number of serious medical conditions such as Parkinson's and Alzheimer's diseases. Studies of short duration (6–12 weeks) have produced contradictory results in randomized clinical trials.[16–19] However, a study lasting over 6 years and involving more than 3000 individuals over the age of 75 who had normal cognition or mild cognitive impairment failed to prevent dementia from all causes or from Alzheimer's disease with standardized ginkgo or placebo.[20]

Drug category and indications for use
Ginkgo biloba may be helpful in preventing memory loss. It may also help to relieve pain associated with claudication (impaired circulation that causes pain when walking).[21]

Mode of action

The flavone glycosides and terpene lactones present in ginkgo may increase blood supply to tissues through their ability to reduce the viscosity of blood and cause vasodilatation.[17]

Warnings and precautions

Bleeding has been reported with the use of ginkgo, and excessive bleeding may occur if an individual is taking anticoagulant drugs such as aspirin or warfarin. Indiviuals taking anticoagulant drugs should consult a physician before using ginkgo. Individuals may experience headache and nausea.

Recommended doses

Adults may take 80–240 mg of standardized ginkgo leaf extract two to three times a day. Gingko is not recommended for those under 18 years of age. The standardized extract (EGb-761) contains 24–45% flavone glycosides and 6% terpine lactones.[21]

Products

Ginkoba and many generic formulations.

Coronary heart disease

Coronary heart (artery) disease (CHD) is a major cause of morbidity and death in the USA. Risks factors such as age, gender, and family history cannot be controlled, but obesity, high serum lipids, and smoking may be controlled or modified. A healthy diet, moderate exercise, and no smoking are behaviors that can reduce the risk of CHD. The American Heart Association and the American Dietetic Association recommend reducing saturated animals fats in the daily diet and increasing polyunsaturated fats (PUFAs) obtained from certain fish (salmon, mackerel, herring, trout, sardine, and tuna), nuts and seeds (walnuts, flaxseed), and plant oils (soy and canola).[22,23] These foods contain omega-3 fatty acids (eicosapentaenoic acid (EPA) and docosahexaenoic acid (DHA)).

The FDA recommended that individuals increase omega-3 fatty acids in their diets, and also permitted dietary supplements EPA and DHA to claim that their use may reduce the risk of CHD.[24] Both EPA and DHA are available in higher concentrations than permitted in OTC dietary supplements in a prescription drug, omega-3-acid ethyl esters (Lovaza), for the treatment of high serum triglycerides.

Omega-3 fatty acids

Drugs and indications for use

Omega-3 fatty acids (fish oils) may reduce the risk of CHD.

Mode of action

Omega-3 fatty acids reduce levels of triglycerides, decrease platelet adhesion, decrease sympathetic nervous system overactivity (vasoconstriction), reduce inflammation associated with arachidonic acid-derived mediators, reduce insulin resistance, and may decease ventricular arrhythmias.[23,25]

Warnings and precautions

Individuals who are taking anticoagulant drugs or who have bleeding problems should consult a physician before using omega-3 products. Individuals may experience a fishy taste and may have diarrhea.

Recommended dose

There is no specific recommendation for the daily amount of omega-3 fatty acids. However, the FDA recommends that adults and those over 18 years of age should not take more than 2000 mg of EPA and DHA daily.[24] Formulations based on FDA's standard for menhaden fish contain 1000 mg of fish oil that has 180 mg EPA and 120 mg DHA. Concentrated formulations of fish oil products contain twice the amount of EPA and DHA.

The American Heart Association recommends that individuals without risk factors eat two servings (3 ounces (80 g) per serving) of fish per week, and those who have risk factors should eat four servings of fish per week.[22] The American Heart Association also recommends that not more than 3000 mg of fish oil supplements be taken daily without consulting a physician.

Products

Omega-3 fish oils are available from many generic manufacturers.

Case study exercises

Case 1 A young woman who has discussed the use Alli for weight loss with the pharmacist is getting ready to leave the pharmacy. She asks the pharmacist if there is anything else she needs to do to successfully complete the scheduled weight-loss program.

The pharmacist asks if she has any vitamin products at home that contain vitamins A, D, E, and K. Alli will prevent the absorption of these fat-soluble vitamins and they must be replaced in the diet. These vitamins should be taken every evening as long as she uses Alli.

Case 2 HY is a 59-year-old man who has been smoking two packs of cigarettes a day for 20 years. He has decided to stop smoking and doesn't want to use any gum or lozenges because he is having extensive periodontal dental work done. He asks the pharmacist to recommend a product.

The pharmacist recommends that he use the dermal patch system for his nicotine replacement program. He should use begin with the high dose, the 21 mg patch, and follow the directions for tapering in the product's instructions. The pharmacist suggests that he consider joining a smoking cessation program because individuals in these programs tend to have greater success when they have a support group.

Case 3 MJ asks the pharmacist why the glucosamine tablets she bought last week and has taken for 5 days did not help relieve her arthritis pain.
The pharmacist explains that glucosamine helps to increase growth of cartilage tissue in the joints and that it may take a month or more before it exerts its maximum effect. She should continue taking 1500 mg of glucosamine daily and if she has pain she should take acetaminophen. If she feels no improvement after taking glucosamine for 4 to 6 weeks, she may decide to stop taking it. She could also consult her doctor if the pain becomes worse.

Case 4 MR, a 49-year-old woman, asks the pharmacist if she should use 5% minoxidil because she is beginning to lose hair on the crown of her head.
The hair loss MR described fits that of male pattern baldness, androgenic alopecia. She may want to try using minoxidil 2% solution, but should not use minoxidil 5% because is not approved for use by women.

Case 5 KN is a 56-year-old man who had a stroke and is taking a baby aspirin daily as prescribed by his doctor. He tells the pharmacist that he is getting forgetful and wants to know if ginkgo will help him.
The pharmacist tells KN that some clinical studies show positive results of ginkgo in preventing memory loss when compared with a placebo, while other studies show no effect. However, ginkgo increases the risk of excessive bleeding in individuals who are taking anticoagulant drugs like aspirin. The pharmacist recommends that KN consult his doctor about this situation before he takes any ginkgo product.

References

1. *Final Rule Declaring Dietary Supplements Containing Ephedrine Alkaloids Adulterated Because They Present an Unreasonable Risk.* Rockville, MD: US Department of Health and Human Services, Food and Drug Administration, 2004: 1–363. www.fda.gov/OHRMS/DOCKETS/98fr/1995n-0304-nfr0001.pdf (accessed March 4, 2009).
2. Bent S *et al.* Safety and efficacy of *citrus aurantium* for weight loss. *Am J Cardiol* 2004; 94: 1359–1361.

3. *Orlistat Information.* www.fda.gov/cder/drug/infopage/orlistat_otc/ (accessed March 4, 2009).
4. *Treating Tobacco Use and Dependence: 2008 Update.* www.ahrq.gov/path/tobacco.htm (accessed March 12, 2009).
5. Corelli RL, Hudman KS. Tobacco use and dependence. In: Koda-Kimble MA *et al.* eds. *Applied Therapeutics: The Clinical Use of Drugs,* 9th edn. Philadelphia, PA: Wolters Kluwer Lippincott Williams & Wilkins, 2009: 85-1–89-30.
6. Fiore MC *et al. Treating Tobacco Use and Dependence. Quick Reference Guide for Clinicians.* Rockville, MD: US Department of Health and Human Services, Public Health Service, 2000. www.surgeongeneral.gov/tobacco/tobaqrg.htm (accessed May 28, 2009).
7. Buys LM, Elliott E. Osteoarthritis. In: DiPiro JT *et al.* eds. *Pharmacotherapy: A Pathophysiologic Approach,* 7th edn. New York: McGraw Hill, 2008: 1519–1550.
8. *Dietary Supplements Glucosamine and/or Chondroitin Fare No Better Than Placebo in Slowing Structural Damage of Knee Osteoarthritis.* www.nih.gov/news/newsletter/2009_january/gait.htm (accessed March 13, 2009).
9. Jellin JM *et al.* Glucosamine hydrochoride. In: *Pharmacist's Letter/Prescriber's Letter Natural Medicines Comprehensive Database,* 3rd edn. Stockton, CA: Therapeutic Research Faculty; 2000: 492–496.
10. *Product Review: Joint Supplements (Glucosamine, Chrondroitin, and MSM).* www.consumerLab.com (accessed March 12, 2009).
11. Otberg N *et al.* Androgenic alopecia. *Endrinol Metab Clin North Am* 2007; 36: 379–398.
12. *Guidance for Industry Labeling OTC Human Drug Products Updating Labeling in ANDAs.* www.fda.gov/cder/guidance/3954dft.htm (accessed March 31, 2009).
13. Rogaine. www.Rogaine.com (accessed March 31, 2009).
14. *Ginseng (American ginseng, Asian ginseng, Chinese ginseng, Korean red ginseng,* Panax ginseng: Panax *spp. including* P. ginseng, C.C.Meyer *and* P. quinquefolius L., *excluding* Eleutherococcus senticosus*).* www.nlm.nih.gov/medlineplus/druginfo/natural/patient-ginseng.html (accessed May 27, 2009).
15. Asian ginseng. http://nccam.nih.gov/asianginseng.html (accessed May 27, 2009).
16. Solomon PR *et al.* Ginkgo for memory enhancement: a randomized controlled trial. *JAMA* 2002; 288: 835–840.
17. Birks J. *Ginkgo biloba* for cognitive impairment and dementia. *Cochrane Database Syst Rev* 2007; (2): CD003120.
18. Mix JA. An examination of the efficacy of *Ginkgo biloba* extract EGb761 on the neuropsychologic functioning of cognitively intact older adults. *J Alt Complement Med* 2000; 6: 219–229.
19. van Dongen MC *et al.* The efficacy of ginkgo for elderly people with dementia and age-associated memory impairment: new results of a randomized clinical trial. *J Am Geriatr Soc* 2000; 48: 1183–1194.
20. DeKosky ST *et al.* Ginkgo biloba for prevention of dementia: a randomized controlled trial. *JAMA* 2008; 300: 2253–2262.
21. *Ginkgo (*Ginkgo biloba L.*).* www.nlm.nih.gov/medlineplus/druginfo/natural/patient-ginkgo.html (accessed May 27, 2009).
22. *Fish and Omega-3 Fatty Acids.* http://216.185.112.5/presenter.jhtml?identifier=4632 (accessed May 30, 2009).
23. van Horn L *et al.* The evidence for dietary prevention and treatment of cardiovascular disease. *J Am Diet Assoc* 2008; 108: 287–331.
24. *Omega-3 Fatty Acids and Coronary Heart Disease.* [Docket No. 2003Q-0401.] www.fda.gov/Drugs/ResourcesForYou/Consumers/ucm073992.html#omega3 (accessed June 1, 2009).
25. DeFilippis AP, Sperling LS. Understanding omega-3's. *Am Heart J* 2006; 151: 564–570.

Index